Pregnancy and Birth

pleasures and problems

Christopher Macy
and
Frank Falkner

HARPER & ROW, PUBLISHERS
New York   Hagerstown   Philadelphia
San Francisco   London   Sydney

This book was devised and produced
by Multimedia Publications Inc

General Editor: *Dr. Leonard Kristal*
Prod Mgr/Art Dir/Design: *Bob Vari*
Picture Researcher: *Judy Kristal*
Illustrator: *Diana Sherman*

Compilation copyright ©
Multimedia Publications Inc Willemstad (Curaçao) 1979
Text copyright © Christopher Macy and Frank Falkner 1979
All rights reserved

First published in Holland 1979 by
Multimedia Publications Inc

British Library Cataloguing in Publication Data
Macy, Christopher
Falkner, Frank
    Pregnancy and Birth: pleasures and problems
    References pg. 120–124
    Includes index
ISBN 06 384741 8   paper

Colour origination: United Artists Ltd, Israel
Typeset by CCC and printed by William Clowes & Sons Limited
Beccles and London

Contents

I

The background to pregnancy

The birth of a child has been called 'an everyday miracle'. It is commonplace, yet a process of such complexity that it is far beyond any artificial human accomplishment. Pregnancy, too, is commonplace, and yet psychologically speaking it is still a mystery for most of us. Strangely enough, the nature and process of pregnancy is still a new frontier, although psychologists and other scientists have investigated the mechanism of learning, the forces of social behaviour, the dynamics of business and industry and have made great strides in therapy and personal growth. So new is much of the work that is described in the following pages that it has never before been published to be read by mothers-to-be, women in general, and their husbands.

A pregnant woman does not sit passively, nor even carry on her old life untouched while the new baby grows within her. She must make a number of very major psychological adaptations. First, there is the adaptation to that new life within her, something that is part of her, yet separate from her. Secondly,

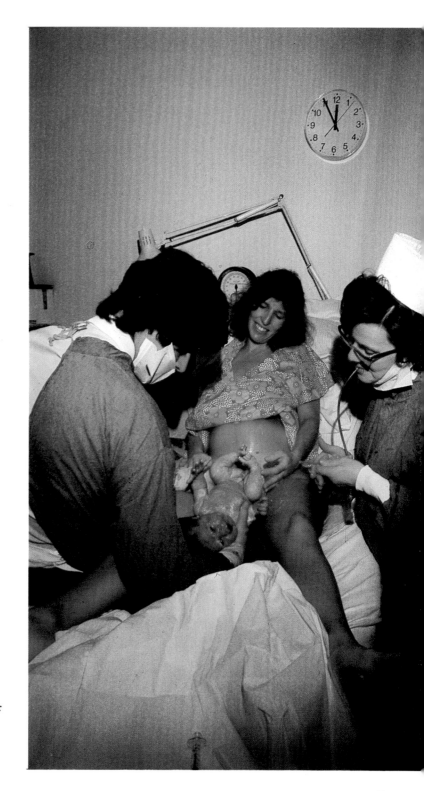

The 'everyday miracle':
for mother and
child the radical
beginning to a new
kind of life.

5

there is the change in her status from un-mother to mother, a change that many psychologists regard as far more important than any other change in life, whether it be puberty, the menopause or marriage. This change means a renegotiation of her relationships with her husband, her own mother and her father, as well as the rest of the society within which she moves. The facts of pregnancy and birth also bring her to a practical awareness of the extraordinary potential of her body. Whether or not she welcomes this knowledge, it certainly needs adjusting to.

This book will consider some of the changes that take place in a mother-to-be and her husband. But in order to understand those changes, we must first look at the biological, social and cultural background against which every pregnancy is set. Different people put different interpretations upon the same event when it happens to them.

Social attitudes

Social attitudes today towards women and motherhood are confused, to say the least. A woman is bombarded by contrary advice and opinion from every side. The influence of psychiatrists like John Bowlby[1] and Renée Spitz[2] has emphasised the vital and irreplaceable role of the mother in the first months and years of a baby's life. Some sections of the women's movement, however, appear to be saying that motherhood is a denigration and denial of human potential. Statements like 'women are denied person-hood' are made in reaction to the expectation that most women will remain at home and give the majority of their time for a few years to the care of their children.

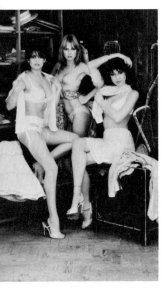

Does this advertisement degrade women? It certainly exploits men—and promotes an idea of feminity that is inimical to maternity.

The women's movement has also produced stickers to be applied to advertisements of a certain kind, saying 'this advertisement exploits women': the idea is that such advertisements portray women as a kind of pleasure machine for men—as sex objects. The possibility is ignored that the same women may be treating the men as pleasure machines, and are quite capable of taking care of themselves in the manipulation of the sexual environment. It would be truer to say that many advertisements in women's magazines today show the kind of women revealed in Aldous Huxley's prophetic novel *Brave New World*; they can eye a man and say, in terms that until recently we recognised only in men: 'Have you had him yet?' 'No, I think I might have him tonight!'

Such attitudes betoken a sexual freedom that does not *have* to manifest itself in warring between the sexes or in promiscuity. It can lead to a more open and honest relationship between partners, which must be welcome. But it can also cause women to distrust, even reject the role of motherhood, including the biological functions of birth and suckling. That kind of attitude is little short of disastrous for women, for their husbands and for their future children.

There is, however, another element in such media images that rightly attracts the wrath of women activists. It is an image that is a modern survival of past attitudes, stripped down, cleaned up, polished and intensified. We refer, of course, to the image of the helpless female.

Her history has been mixed, but it may be that she never wielded more influence than now. Perhaps it is because she has come to represent youth as well. The image that stares at us from every quarter today is of a slim eighteen-year-old, unmarried, with all the boys in pursuit, or hanging on the arm of one, gambolling on beaches, in sports cars, in the bright spots, and just occasionally in the countryside.

Danger in stereotypes

Today 'feminine' has come to mean something very special, and this could represent a new trap for women. Many of the studies that have been done with pregnant women report that those with problems tend to owe them, at least in part, to a difficulty in accepting their feminine role. It used to be taken for granted that the feminine role should culminate in motherhood. This is no longer so—at least in the eyes of some powerful public image-makers. A girl or an older woman is 'feminine' if she is lithe, spry and ready to be courted. To Edwardian forebears the feminine woman was the one with a small waist and flaring curves to large breasts and large hips, betokening her readiness and ability to bear children, or, better still, her actually having borne two or three. Today our conception of femininity demands an altogether leaner, younger, more boyish shape.

Perhaps we need two concepts. The French psychoanalyst P. C. Racamier has proposed two words, one for biological motherhood and one for psychological motherhood. And American psychologist Niles Newton has drawn a distinction between 'cultural femininity' and 'biological femininity'. We might perhaps use the word 'feminine' for the woman who is eternally young (or who strives to be) and is untouched by her own biology, whether it involves sex, childbearing or ordinary ageing. The word 'female' would denote the woman who accepts the implications for her lifestyle of her biology and biological functions.

One British study by Michael Humphrey[3] shows that some women make precisely this distinction in their own thinking, although they are not necessarily conscious of doing so. To the group of women that he studied 'feminine' meant young and sexually attractive. Motherhood and femininity did not go together for these women, nor did motherhood and sexual attractiveness. In fact they nicely showed up the nonsensical paradox in our present cultural thinking: the more 'motherly' a woman, the less 'attractive' she is, and therefore the less likely to marry and have children. On the other hand, the more psychologically unprepared for childbirth, the more likely a woman is to enter into a contract, marriage, with the probable outcome of having children. (Interestingly, the men in this study did not make a similar split in thinking about themselves. To them fatherhood and masculinity meant the same thing.)

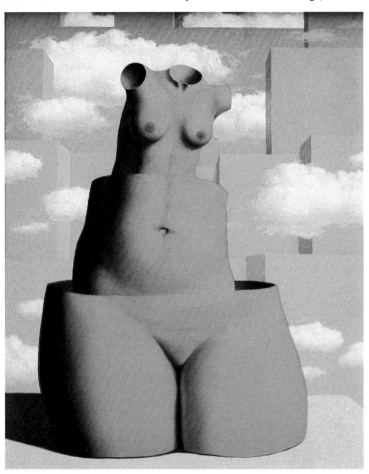

The ideal of 'femininity' is a hollow model for the femaleness of motherhood.

The problem about making this simple division is that it does not allow for those women who are neither predatory sex objects (passive or active) nor mothers, but who reach independent status as persons through work or a career. So perhaps, after all, we need three concepts or words. Better still, we should simply recognise the various factors pulling in different directions on a woman who is considering becoming a mother or who has actually started a pregnancy. The important thing is not the shape of a woman, nor how attractive or young she is, nor whether she is a career woman—but whether or not she accepts her own femaleness, sexually and reproductively. Niles Newton found that women who aimed for the cultural definition of femininity were less happy with their pregnancy than those who felt more biologically female. In the terms we are suggesting, femaleness culminates in motherhood, while femininity actually leads away from it.

Richard and Katherine Gordon[4] found that intellectual doubt and conflict about the role of women and of mothers can produce emotional problems in pregnant women regardless of their own personal psychological histories. An experiment in psychological preparation aimed at preventing or counteracting role conflict resulted in significantly fewer emotional upsets during pregnancy and led to mothers' being healthier mentally and physically four to six years later.

Other societies

For most women an important transition is the psychological shift from youthful 'femininity'—whether predatory or dependent—to the state of resourceful and dependable mother. In societies other than those of Western Europe and America life is simpler for both men and women. This is not to say that these other societies all present the same picture. The variety of social patterns throughout the whole of humanity is immense. Take, for example, one small area in New Guinea that the anthropologist Margaret Mead and her husband, Gregory Bateson, studied. Within a few miles, spread out along the banks of the Sepik river, live four tribes. They are separated by distances no greater than those commuted by many Europeans and Americans every day, yet there are important differences in the roles occupied by men and women. Among the Iatmul and Tchambuli, men and women have separate secret societies and very different social roles. An Iatmul mother treats her baby after only a few weeks as an emotional equal, with a will of his own. She stops carrying him about and leaves him until he is crying vigorously before she picks him up and feeds him, which she then does generously. Tchambuli mothers carry their babies longer and feed them more readily. If an Iatmul mother has an argument with a small child, she may chase him round the house with a paddle, treating him almost as she would an equal with whom she had a quarrel. A Tchambuli mother simply tucks him under her arm, accepting his dependence.

The Mundugumor, by contrast, have come as near as is possible to destroying any difference between the sexes. The women have adopted what we would call masculine attitudes. They enjoy sex but hate the consequences. Pregnancy is a disaster, and many women adopt children rather than bear them themselves. A Mundugumor mother carries her baby in a harsh basket high on her back, as far away from the breast as possible. She nurses him standing up, ceasing as soon as there is a hint that the child has had enough, and weans him early and hard. Among the Arapesh, though there is a formal separation of men's and women's cultures, in practice the two sexes lead nearly identical lives. Both cherish their children. An Arapesh mother carries her baby in a soft cloth bag slung from a band round her forehead

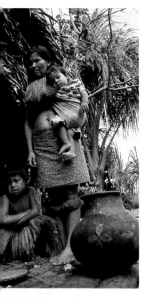

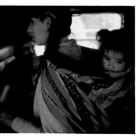

The variety of social patterns is immense.

9

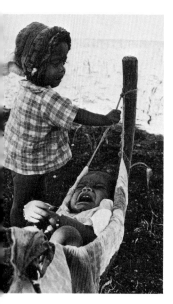

Other people's child care: babies in India look after one another while mothers cultivate.

and feeds him frequently, offering the breast even when it is not asked for, watching her child's feeding with gentle interest.

Different as these four societies are from each other, within each one there is a consistency. Even allowing for differences in individual character, the behaviour that is expected from male and female, from mothers and fathers, is clear. The rules may not be simple, but they are thoroughly taught by each generation to the succeeding one. There may be an abrupt change for a boy at puberty—as there is for boys in many societies—but his new place as a man is taught to him in elaborate initiation ceremonies that may go on for weeks. Both boys and girls (whose progression to adulthood is smoother and easier) learn much from simply observing everyday life in their small, intimate and open societies. Children take part in work, sex play and child care from an early age. Even if their theories about how the world works and how the human body functions are in our eyes 'incorrect', their practical knowledge is more extensive and more secure.

When a couple from a 'primitive' village continue to make love enthusiastically throughout a pregnancy because they believe that a baby is formed out of a mingling of semen and menstrual blood, they are acting in ignorance of the scientific facts of physiology. They are secure however in their knowledge of what they believe to be true, their own version of the 'facts'. In Western society, one of the commonest questions that pregnant couples ask is, 'Is it all right to make love during pregnancy?' They, too, are ignorant of the physiological facts, but lack anything else to put in their place. And out of that ignorance comes anxiety.

Hidden pregnancy

In societies like those we have described, pregnancy and birth are a clearly visible part of the life-cycle. In the West, even as late as the 1950s, many of the illustrations used in pregnancy manuals did not show pregnant women. The swelling of the belly was seen as an embarrassment. Many pregnancy garments for women, while they acknowledged publicly that a pregnant woman was something special, tended tactfully to conceal her condition. In fact the smock so successfully disguised the form of the woman's body that many a woman has been taken for pregnant just because she is wearing a smock—no other evidence being visible.

Contrast this with the open recognition of pregnancy in other societies. Margaret Mead writes:

The little girl . . . also sees pregnancy treated with the greatest openness and simplicity. Childbirth itself may be shrouded from all but adult eyes . . . but nowhere in any of these societies is pregnancy concealed, and indeed it requires heavy clothing and shuttered houses and an economic system that can withdraw women from almost all productive work, to make it possible to conceal pregnancy from the eyes of the world . . . 'I Wajan is pregnant, some day you will be pregnant. My!

what a fat little tummy you have! Perhaps you are pregnant now?' In Bali little girls between two and three walk with purposely thrust out little bellies, and the older women tap them as they pass. 'Pregnant', they tease. So the little girl knows that although the signs of her membership of her own sex are slight, her breasts mere buttons no bigger than her brothers', her genitals a simple inconspicuous fold, some day she will be pregnant, some day she will have a baby.

Our own society is changing. Photographs in women's magazines now tend to emphasise the bulge as a dramatic event. At the same time, these photographs distort reality in another way. They are a novel extension of the glamour photographer's work. So pregnant women are shown as elegantly slim—apart from that interesting bulge—and radiantly at peace with themselves and their state. Indeed, you will rarely see a photograph of a pregnant woman doing the housework, going shopping or changing the nappies or diapers on an older child. One might imagine that pregnant women are rarely indoors but live entirely in beautiful gardens and parks. Such pictures rightly emphasise the importance of the private inner experience of pregnancy—but in a limited way, leaving out of account the everyday social and working world in which a pregnant woman moves.

The bulge: dramatic, but not glamorous or convenient—and women's work is still never done!

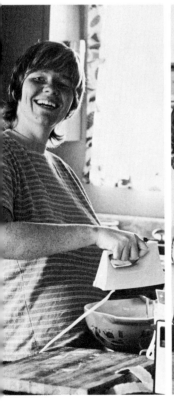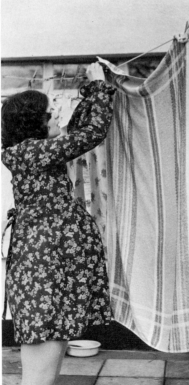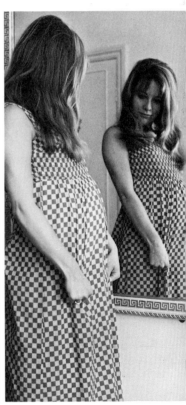

The legacy of our past

We have inherited our attitudes from our forebears, and it makes them easier to understand if we know a little about our own history. For our ancestors pregnancy was most of the time an event to be feared. People today under the age of forty or so can have little idea of how hard life was for most people in Europe and America until the Second World War. One woman interviewed by one of the authors regretted having only one child, born in 1947. 'But things was different then,' she said, 'times was hard.' Even then life was rich compared with the conditions endured during the nineteenth century with the flight to the cities, new frontiers in the USA, successive agricultural slumps. In earlier centuries there were regular times of hardship to the point of famine.

In such circumstances different cultures adapt in different ways. Some, such as the Arapesh, cope well and retain a caring society. Others become harsh and punitive. In Europe and Britain the age of marriage rose and fell with the state of the economy. In many periods men and women did not marry and bear children until well into their thirties.[5] Given the basic biological drive to procreate, the social environmental controls imposed in order to achieve population control by this means must have been stringent.

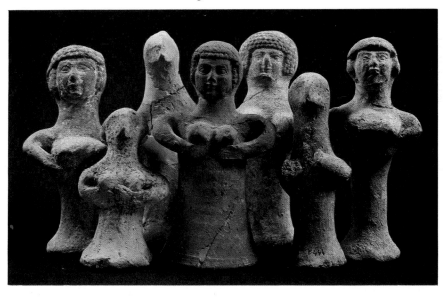

Ancient symbols of womanhood stressed their reproductive and nourishing roles.

In many societies girls are able to have intercourse freely without conceiving until they choose their life partners, marry and settle down, when the natural sequence of conception and childbearing begins. European women lacked this skill—or rather tended to use it in an inefficient way. In Europe abstinence was the only safe means of contraception. And since marriage was ordained by the Church as being primarily for the begetting of children, abstinence was frowned upon in marriage.

Illegitimate children were a challenge to the economic stability of the family and society. And even within marriage, many more children were born than could be supported economically. Thomas Coram founded his hospitals for foundlings because he saw so many children abandoned and dying on rubbish heaps and in sewers in eighteenth-century London.

Creating a taboo around sex was an understandable strategy to try to keep to a minimum the number of children born. For women the penalty of bearing a child out of wedlock could be banishment, ending in death. We tend to think of the disapproval of unmarried mothers as rooted in Victorian prudery. But the Victorians did not invent puritanism; social control of sexual activity has a long history in the severity and misery of poverty.

Another factor that influenced European and hence American attitudes to women and childbearing was religion. Attitudes to love, sex, pregnancy and childbirth in Europe and America cannot be separated from the historical teachings of the Christian Church. These were not simple. Even the most fervent non-believer must surely admit that the marriage service in the Anglican Book of Common Prayer is a moving human document, with its words, put into the mouth of the new husband, 'With my body I thee worship.' But against this must be set the doctrine of the Virgin Birth. The ideal woman—the person who, for most Christians, sits at the side of God the Son and intercedes for humanity's sins—bore her son when she was a virgin.

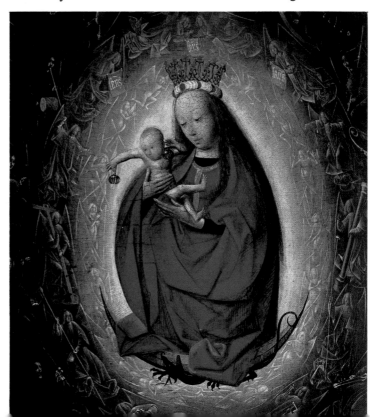

The dragon at the bottom of the womblike enclosure of the Virgin reinforces the message: 'This child was not conceived in sin . . .'

The idealisation of women has been a strong undercurrent in Western society. In the Middle Ages the ideal was courtly love— a love which was never consummated. The knight did not woo, win and wed his heart's desire, but loved and worshipped her from afar. In many societies women are expected to be virgins when they marry. It is still the custom in some Islamic societies for a new husband to show a blood-stained cloth on the morning after the wedding as proof of his prowess and his wife's virtue. Even among the easy-going Samoans, known for their permissiveness for girls before marriage, each village's head girl must be a virgin by proxy for all the others at her own marriage. She, too, has to produce a blood-stained cloth; since she is often not in fact a virgin, she may resort to chicken's blood for effect. Only in Christian society, however, is virginity held up as an ideal for *all* women.

The great anthropologist, Malinowski,[6] described how this ideal still affected European women before the Second World War.

'In modern Europe [among] the orthodox Jewish communities of Poland . . . a pregnant woman is an object of real veneration, and feels proud of her condition. In the Christian Aryan societies, however, pregnancy among the lower classes is made a burden, and regarded as a nuisance; among the well-to-do people it is a source of embarrassment, discomfort and temporary ostracism from ordinary social life.'

In Victorian England people could not bring themselves to identify pregnancy publicly: it was far too embarrassing. Instead, a woman was said to be in an 'interesting condition'.

Childbirth in history

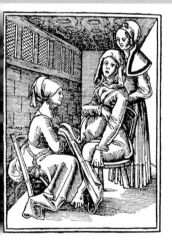

No wonder midwifery was a 'mystery'!

There is a tendency to hark back to a golden past when childbirth was natural and simple, before modern life broke up the family and hospitals took over the care of mother and newborn child. While some aspects of pregnancy and birth were probably better managed, others were not. (It is interesting to note in passing that the word 'nostalgia' was coined in the nineteenth century to denote a neurotic condition.)

In the first manual for midwives, published in English in 1540, the author or publisher felt it necessary to apologise for the publication. The prologue states: 'Many thinke it not meete ne fitting that such matters be intreated of so plainly in our mother and vulgar language to the dishonour of womanhood and the derision of their secrets.' A century later another such text omitted any description or drawings of 'the parts destined to generation' as not being 'absolutely necessary'—this in a text for midwives!

The embarrassment expressed in the prologue of the manual for midwives may have been representative of the feelings of the

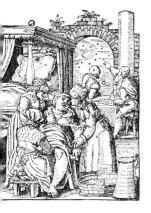

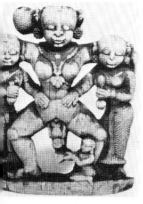

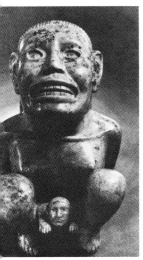

The good old days?
Birth stool, delivery
astride or agonised
squat gave
childbirth a bad name.

newly emerging middle class. It reflected the fact that the printer must have been a man, putting into print material which would, for the first time, become available to other men.

Women at this time almost certainly had their own subculture. The 'secrets' that the author referred to would have been the secrets of women in general, not just the privacy of individual females. Material on historical folkways is hard to gather. But we know that, among the rural population, the old pagan religions did not entirely die out in Europe until the middle of the eighteenth century. Traditional folk skills in such matters as medicine and childbirth must have been increasingly taken over at that time by the Christian middle classes. Male midwives arrived in the first half of the eighteenth century and played an increasingly large part. Then the doctors saw a convenient division of labour between male doctors and female midwives, and male midwives were outlawed again.

What can it have been like to be pregnant and give birth in the Middle Ages? Those accounts that have come down to us are scarcely trustworthy, partly because the authors of most accounts were men who can never have been present at a birth, and partly because many such accounts are framed in the magical terms of the period. Many writers were simply not concerned with the physical or psychological welfare of mother and child, but only with their spiritual state. Most women were quite untouched by the limited amount of obstetric and paediatric knowledge then available. Before scientific medicine, that cannot have been anything but an advantage. One Dauphine of France (the wife of the heir to the throne) was in labour for 30 hours during which she was bled at regular intervals. When the baby girl was finally delivered, she was wrapped in a lambskin freshly flayed from a live animal in the lying-in room. Since sleep after a difficult birth was held to be dangerous the Dauphine was kept awake forcibly for some hours. Then her room was sealed and she was left in complete darkness for nine days.[7]

In the twelfth century one writer deplored the Irish habit of leaving babies unswathed and neglecting the cruelties practised elsewhere. 'Their tender limbs are not helped by frequent baths or formed by any useful art,' he wrote. 'The midwives do not use hot water to raise the nose or press down the face or lengthen the legs. *Unaided nature* according to her own judgement arranges and disposes without the help of any art the limbs that she has produced.' (Our italics.)

In one respect mothers and babies were better off than in our more immediate past. During the early Middle Ages some statues of the Virgin and Child showed her breast-feeding the infant Jesus. Bartholomew of England taught that since the mother's blood had nourished the child in the womb, her milk was the best food for him after birth. He also realised the psychological importance of breast-feeding, because, 'The mother loves her own child most tenderly, embraces it and kisses it, nurses and cares for it most solicitously.'

How we feel about children

'Make every child a wanted child' ran a slogan during the sixties and seventies. While the campaign had perfectly worthy aims, the slogan reinforces a common idea that is seriously oversimplified. It makes a sharp distinction between the 'wanted' and the 'unwanted' child. In many pregnancies, however, probably even in most, things are not so clear-cut.[8]

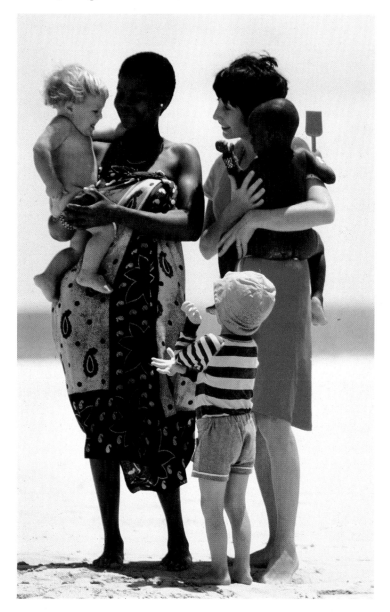

It may look as if the experiences are interchangeable—but there are as many attitudes to pregnancy, birth and childrearing as there are cultures.

Our attitudes to children have evolved over the two-and-a-half thousand years or so of our civilisation, so that an ever-increasing value is placed on our children and their happiness. *The History of Childhood* by Lloyd de Mause[9] shows that a strong current of hostility towards children has prevailed throughout recorded history. Not only were unwanted babies put out to die, left to starve or deliberately overlain and smothered in bed; but those that survived were commonly treated in quite astonishingly barbarous ways.

De Mause believes that child rearing has evolved slowly over the last two thousand years through certain stages. In antiquity, infanticide typifies the position of children: they had to fight to survive against a hostile adult world. By the Middle Ages, parents accepted that children had a right to live, but most were themselves too immature to care for them properly. With the Renaissance, and the explosion of Humanist learning in the fifteenth and sixteenth centuries, came an ambivalent phase, with parents wishing to care for their children but seeing in them the form of the devil. From the eighteenth century onwards, according to de Mause the 'intrusive stage' developed, as more mature adults felt able to cope with active child management.

As the quality of child care improved, the death rate dropped. The nineteenth century saw the 'socialisation phase', which reflected the new moral approach to all human welfare. Life (for the middle classes, at least) had ceased to be such a struggle, and the claims of children were taken seriously. The last phase portrayed by de Mause, which is only now in its early stages, accepts that the child is a human being in his own right, who in many respects knows far better than any adult what is good for him. The task of parents is not to impose a stereotype of good behaviour on the child but to allow him to establish his own character and path through life.

The love and care that we Western parents ideally bestow on our children, and the combination of freedom and guidance that we allow them, place responsibilities on us that parents in earlier generations did not know. To hark back to a mythical golden age is, therefore, not only to look for something that never existed, but to miss the point of the challenge that faces today's new parents. We want a better experience and outcome of pregnancy than our ancestors. If we pay as much attention to the psychology involved as we have to the biology, then we cannot fail to make life better for both mothers and their children.

2 The experience of pregnancy

Our history has left us with a wide range of different ideas about what happens in pregnancy, and what it means to a woman and her husband. Added to them are the different theories that have emerged out of psychological and sociological studies over the last hundred years. Each woman probably forms her ideas about her own pregnancy, out of a mixture of those she meets in reading and talking to other mothers and professionals concerned with her care. No two women are likely to have exactly the same ideas and emotions.

How a woman and her husband experience pregnancy together depends to a very large extent on their previous ideas about pregnancy, childbirth and the baby that results. Depending on this, the woman's pregnancy can be a joy or a burden, the end or the beginning of a good life, the making or the undoing of the marital relationship.

In this chapter we present a selection of the ideas about pregnancy that are common, some in professional thinking, some in our general culture and some in both. Some carry more weight than others, some are more 'respectable' than others. But all contribute both to a woman's own experience and to the advice she will find offered to her by family, friends and professionals. She might, indeed, have a little fun trying to place her thoughts and what other people say to her into the appropriate category or approach.

Motherhood as instinct

Possibly this is a view more likely to be held by men than by women. In its crudest form it takes the line that just as every man's main purpose in life is to copulate, so every woman is instinctively driven to bear and care for children. Life is simply a merry-go-round driven by the procreative urge.

In a more sophisticated form the view is matched by the theory that there is a set of innate patterns of behaviour that are triggered by events both inside the woman and in her environment.[1] Each of these pieces of behaviour helps to trigger the

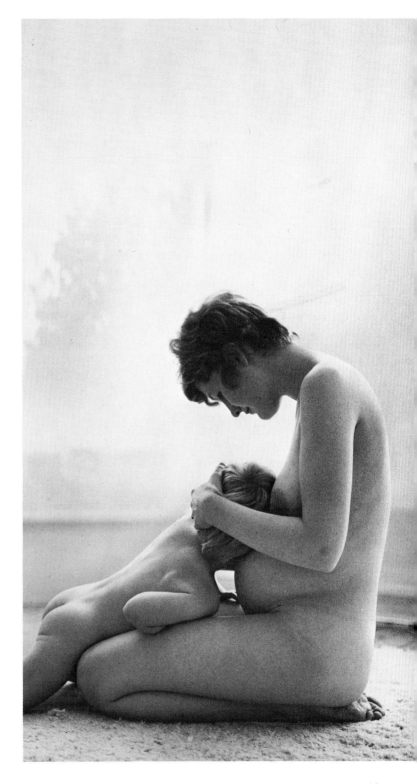

*'What's it feel like,
having a baby
inside your tummy?'*

19

next, so that there is a 'cascade' effect. For men the soft curves of a woman's body and the twin protuberances of breasts and buttocks are said by some ethologists to be 'innate releasing mechanisms' or triggers for men's sexual behaviour. For women the triggers are more subtle. Love and closeness have more effect than visual stimuli. Once she is pregnant the feeling of the child within her, and the experience of birth itself, trigger a state in which the new mother is especially responsive to the child, and in which the presence of the child triggers her to explore and then love the baby.

It's the same the whole world over—some innate behaviour is common to all mammalian births.

Research with animals has demonstrated that much of their behaviour in pregnancy and mothering is innate,[2] but that it can be all too easily disrupted.[3]

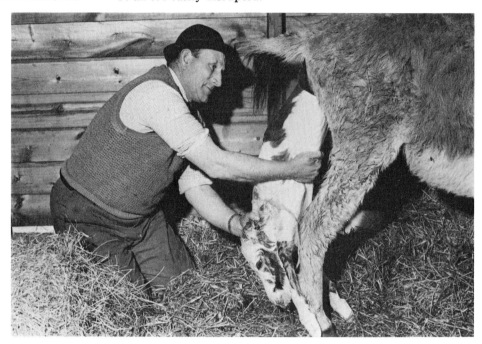

Studies of different human societies show that, despite a variety of cultures, there is a core of behaviour that is constant. We too, it seems, have a basic pattern of behaviour which is extensively shaped and guided by the rules of our different societies, but which runs, like an underground stream, beneath all our attitudes and behaviour.[4, 5]

Pregnancy as promise

Sometimes the mother-to-be is seen as living in a sort of heavenly limbo, in a state of blessed suspension between girlhood and womanhood. She has left the irresponsibilities of idle youth behind, but has yet to take on the responsibilities of maternal maturity. Enough of youth is left to her, however, to enjoy life with the girls just a little longer. If she is lucky enough to be able to give up work early in the pregnancy, she has an opportunity such as never before to lead a life of leisure for a short time, to buy new clothes, to take tea with friends, and perhaps to take in a matinée now and again.

At the same time motherhood is close enough for her to assume just a little of the aura of maternity, of the status of motherhood, to lord it, ever so slightly, over her as yet childless friends and colleagues.

It is a time of suspended animation, when the child that is not yet a child grows within her, the claims he makes on her body and energy unnoticed, at least until the latter stages. 'Vegetative calm' prevails, while growth goes on stealthily, healthily and autonomously, almost accidentally, and she feels so uninvolved.

Birth marks an irrevocable end to this period of temporary absolution, and the beginning of a life of burden.

Pregnancy as illness

Some women see and experience the nine months of pregnancy as nine months of deviation from the norm. For them, before she becomes pregnant for the first time, a woman is a woman and a girl is a girl. After the birth the woman becomes a woman with a child, the girl becomes a girl who has had a baby. Normality has been restored, and with it a little extra. There is a feeling that it is unfair that the old stories about babies being found under very ripe gooseberry bushes or brought by rather gentle storks are not true.

According to this view the swollen legs and ankles, the sickness, the eternal tiredness and the heavily distended belly must be borne with fortitude and then forgotten. Of course it is only natural (in this view) for a woman to be upset, or to be easily distressed. She will probably want to eat all sorts of strange things—coal, carrots, one brand of baked beans and no other— all signs that she really is not quite normal for the time being.

The well meant and eminently sensible advice in guide-books for pregnant women can sometimes be taken by them to reinforce the illness view of pregnancy. 'Pregnancy is often bedevilled by a whole variety of minor ailments ... morning sickness, heartburn, piles and constipation, faintness and dizziness, varicose veins'; 'Visit your doctor or midwife regularly ... listen carefully to the advice your doctor or midwife gives you ... follow doctor's orders.'[6]

Many studies have found that pregnant women go through emotional and personality changes but return to 'normal' after the birth. We shall show later that while women understandably show changes in their psychological characteristics during pregnancy, to say that they return to 'normal' afterwards misses the point of what really happens.

Pregnancy as ordeal

Trial by ordeal, or mediaeval Catch-22: survival conferred a special grace. Some pregnant women feel they have been 'thrown in at the deep end', too.

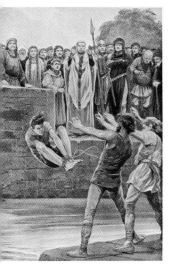

This section might perhaps more properly be headed 'birth as an ordeal', but the attitude embraces both. Birth is the great ordeal that girls must go through in order to prove their womanhood; pregnancy is both part of the ordeal and a preparation for it. There is a heavy current of this in the subculture of women. The hard work, the dangers and the pains of labour are emphasised. Tales are told of dreadful events in the experience of neighbours or friends. The protective attitude of many doctors is dismissed. 'Birth is hell, and don't let them tell you otherwise,' you may hear. (Certainly you will if you are writing a book on pregnancy.)

There is a hint of a rite of passage in this. In many cultures teenage candidates for the status of adult men or women are subjected to rituals designed to horrify, humiliate and hurt them. In the West such rituals were taken from the ambit of popular culture by the establishment of Church and State, and have now largely withered away. Only these faint disordered echoes remain.

Why do they survive? In the Middle Ages a person accused of wrongdoing was sometimes put to trial by ordeal. There is always a feeling that to go through a time of trial and emerge from it is a proof of more than merely the ability to survive. It is taken as evidence of worth, and indeed is held in itself to increase the worth of the person who endures it. Psychological experiments have confirmed that if the entry to a club is made difficult and unpleasant, then membership of that club is subsequently valued much more highly. This is true even if the club is a trivial affair, and membership largely pointless. Nowadays we value children highly and give the comparatively rare event of pregnancy a high status, so, if we refer to a pregnant woman as being 'in the club', are we doing anything more than anticipate her true membership in the prized club of mothers?

Pregnancy as crisis

Crisis in most people's minds means something unpleasant or bad, as in 'economic crisis'. To a psychologist, however, the word is neutral. One psychologist defined a crisis as a call to action that could be occasioned either by a threat or by a promise. It is the challenge presented when the habitual situation is changed or disturbed, or when it is about to be—when our old patterns of behaviour will no longer do. The external crisis produces an internal crisis in which old patterns of thought and living have to be questioned and examined. The American psychiatrist Gerald Caplan[7] calls this stage a state of 'intrapsychic disequilibrium', which is another way of saying instability.

Many crises are caused by good fortune. Unexpectedly winning

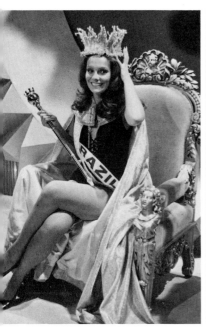

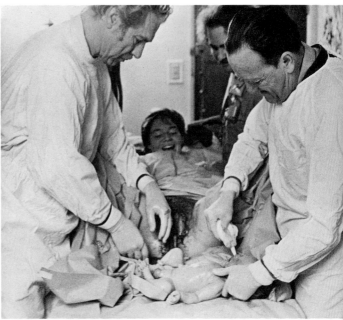

Winning: glad crises of different intensities.

or inheriting a large sum of money produces a crisis in the lives and psychological state of some people.

Many women show an increase in neuroticism during pregnancy, returning to 'normal' after the birth.[8] This reflects their state of disequilibrium as they change psychologically.

Pregnancy as duty

Perhaps this attitude belongs to history. We include it because ripples are probably still present in our society. The great population scare of the 1920s was a declining population. In the English-speaking world the arch proponent of pregnancy as duty was Sir Frederick Truby King, a New Zealand obstetrician. 'Today,' he wrote in 1921, 'our historians and politicians think in terms of regiments and dreadnoughts: the time will come when they must think in terms of babies and motherhood. We must think in such terms too, if we wish Great Britain to be much longer great.'[9] Such attitudes ran through the whole of the Western world at that time: Truby King spoke for a generation, not merely a nation.

The scare of the 1960s and 1970s by contrast, has been over population. In America, where such social movements tend to take greater hold and be conducted with greater vigour than elsewhere, the disapproval of couples who had more than two children ('Stop At Two') was tangible; the approval of couples who did their duty by remaining childless, though a little strained perhaps, was none the less present.

23

Pregnancy as a gateway

According to one estimate 80 per cent of the total population and 90 per cent of women become parents. The desire for children is very strong. For most people marriage and children is what life is all about. A marriage without children is not a proper marriage; a couple without children does not constitute a real family. The word family may even be used to *mean* children, in such expressions as 'they haven't got a family', or 'their family has left home'. Couples are most often asked not 'Are you going to have children?' but 'When are you going to have a family?'

Most parents believe that their lives would be worse without children. Existence would be duller, less emotionally fulfilling, and in a very important way, imbued with less meaning. Parents derive great satisfaction from doing things for their children. A common feeling is 'I want to give my child what I didn't

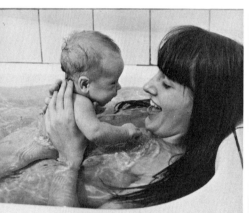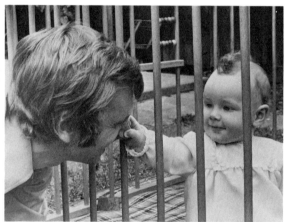

Trivial pleasures make for profound satisfactions in parenthood.

have.'[10,11] It is difficult to say how new these feelings are: they are certainly characteristic of the modern search for a better life both materially and emotionally. Perhaps the feeling that children are a means by which their parents express themselves is stronger in the West than elsewhere in the world. In other cultures, especially those where the extended family is the basis of society, children are valued at least partly because they can keep one in one's old age. In the West, however, the idea of financial dependence on one's adult children is not thought to be right.

For some mothers-to-be whose eyes are fixed on the future, on the role of the mother and the building of a family, the length of a pregnancy comes as something of a shock. The nine months of transition, which for some women flashes by all too quickly, for them becomes an interminable obstruction to what they hoped would be an easy progress from single or young married to motherhood and full adult status.

Pregnancy as growing up

For psychoanalysts as well as for many other men and women pregnancy marks an essential stage in the process of maturing from childhood to full adulthood.[12] Grete Bibring,[13] for example, has portrayed pregnancy and birth as a stage in the life of a woman similar to puberty and the menopause. There is a strong biological underpinning to the psychoanalytical view. The monthly cycle of the woman's body is a process by which her body is repeatedly brought to a state of readiness. If the moment is not taken on the tide, her body rejects the unused ovum and its receptive bed and turns again to the preparation of readiness. Until the tide is taken a woman is not launched on the sea of maturity. She remains as unfulfilled potential only. Psychologically she cannot grow up.

This is the exact opposite of Simone de Beauvoir's assertion that nothing divides men and women except the arbitrary tyranny of an unjust society.[14] The psychoanalytical school takes it that men and women are fundamentally different both biologically and psychologically. But while a man is an adult male simply by virtue of being himself and achieving success in the material world, a girl needs to change in herself before she becomes a woman. Puberty turns a boy into a man, but a girl only into a woman-in-waiting.

Thus when a woman becomes pregnant she is answering a biological call. Her body has been expressing a biological need for motherhood. Pregnancy is the culmination of one stage of the search. If we accept this view, then, as surely as the courtship of animals is 'intended' to reproduce the species, pregnancy is 'intended' by nature to complete the life of women.

Behind much of the social pressure on couples to have children lie views that are different from those of the psychoanalysts only in articulation. 'A different life altogether', one mother said of childless women. 'If they don't want children they should—they just want a good time ...' said another. In the 'good time' suggestion is more than a hint of an accusation of immaturity. Single people and childless couples often also feel that they are regarded with covert pity, in which the suggestion that they are somehow incomplete may be more or less strongly implied.[15]

Such attitudes can produce feelings of anxiety, of being tested, rather than of calm anticipation. Pregnancy is invested with the importance of representing the first appointment with maturity and true adulthood. Many women feel that they are not fully committed to their husbands, nor their husbands to them, until they have had children. Parenthood—rather than an eighteenth or twenty-first birthday, or even than marriage itself—marks the true transition to adulthood.

There is undoubtedly much to support the truth of this idea. At various stages of development in different species, changes in

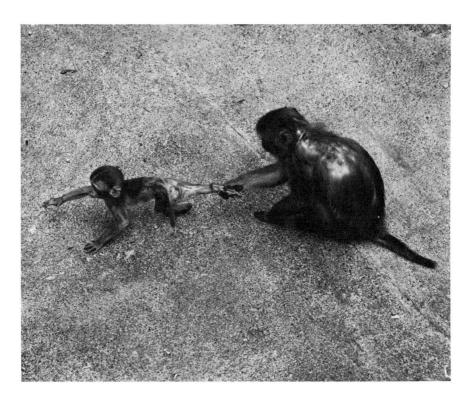

*Next best
to apron strings.*

behaviour are produced by changes in physiology. Many of the growing abilities of baby humans and other animals arise out of the maturation of the nervous system. Growth, too, is not just a process of getting better at more and more things, but involves, in humans, a change in the quality and range of behaviour. At adolescence there are substantial changes in the way young people behave and feel, although how these link with the biological changes that occur in puberty is less clear.

In the same way, it is very likely that the biological processes involved in being pregnant and giving birth, and perhaps in breast-feeding too, produce changes in how a woman behaves and thinks. However, you do not need to be a psychologist to see that some women experience no such change when they become mothers. They do not feel an irresistible surge of love, for the baby or for anyone else, and there is no increase in their caretaking behaviour beyond the mechanical routine, that is inevitably imposed by the responsibility for a new child. So, if there is a link between biological and psychological changes, it is not strong enough to outweigh all other factors.

The idea that motherhood matures a woman in a unique way has an unfortunate secondary implication—that women who remain childless never grow up. Some psychoanalysts go so far as actually to say this. But this is true only if one believes that there is only one path to maturity. Motherhood clearly does mature many women, but, equally, many women who never

26

have children become mature through accepting and carrying out other forms of responsibility—as executives in the business world or looking after other people's children at school, for example.

Perhaps the reader will have noticed something lacking in all these 'models' of pregnancy. None of them seems to take a very positive view of pregnancy itself. The nine months are seen either negatively or as merely the prelude to something positive. Only the model of pregnancy as growing up seems to ascribe any virtue to being pregnant in itself. Even that is pretty negative: pregnancy is good because it responds to a need, because it completes a woman.

In fact there is an element of truth in all the models we have looked at. The positive role of pregnancy can be found by putting them all together.

Pregnancy is an *opportunity* for personal growth.[16] Maturity does not follow automatically from pregnancy and biological motherhood, but it can. The gateway into full adult life via a family will not be passed unless the woman fully adapts to her new task and status. Any minor biomedical upsets will become more than incidental if the mother-to-be is frightened of what lies before her, and ignores what is occurring to her.

Pregnancy is a crisis, because the changes involved are drastic and thorough-going. It is a time when a woman must review both her past and her future. She must compare her ideas about femaleness, femininity and herself, about her mother and her father and what she believes she learned from them, with what she now finds expected of her. If she does not know what is expected of her then that task of comparison and development is made more difficult. Normally, however, the crisis is a benign crisis, with a positive outcome.

Childless, she still takes on some of the responsibilities of parenthood—and some of the pleasures, too.

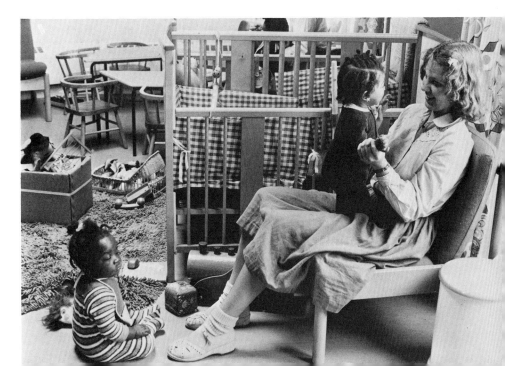

3 The biology of pregnancy

Much of the psychology of pregnancy and the behaviour of the pregnant woman is closely related to the changes that occur in her body. Hence the importance of an understanding of these biomedical changes.

Signs of pregnancy

Most women have an inkling that they are pregnant even before this is confirmed by a doctor. Very rarely a woman who badly wants to become pregnant will imagine she is pregnant and continue to be convinced of this even after medical consultation tells her otherwise, even developing some of the physical signs and feelings of pregnancy. These false or phantom pregnancies need much careful and understanding handling, often by psychiatrists or clinical psychologists.

The first sign of pregnancy is nearly always the 'missed period' or amenorrhea. After an ovum has been fertilised, further ovulation is stopped by hormonal messages. The uterine wall is prepared for implantation of the now fertile ovum. This means that the menstrual cycle ceases. Pregnancy is only one of many possible causes of amenorrhea, so that when amenorrhea occurs in an individual who has irregular menstrual periods this is not a very reliable early sign. However, in women aged 17–39, pregnancy is certainly the most common cause of amenorrhea.

First signs

Breast tissue is very sensitive to hormonal changes and many healthy women experience a feeling of fullness and even some tenderness in their breasts just before menstruation. These changes are related to the female sex hormones oestrogen and progesterone. In early pregnancy, the high levels of these hormones may be a cause of breast tenderness. At the same time there is increased blood supply to the breasts, development of the milk ducts, and enlargement of breast tissue. The nipples become

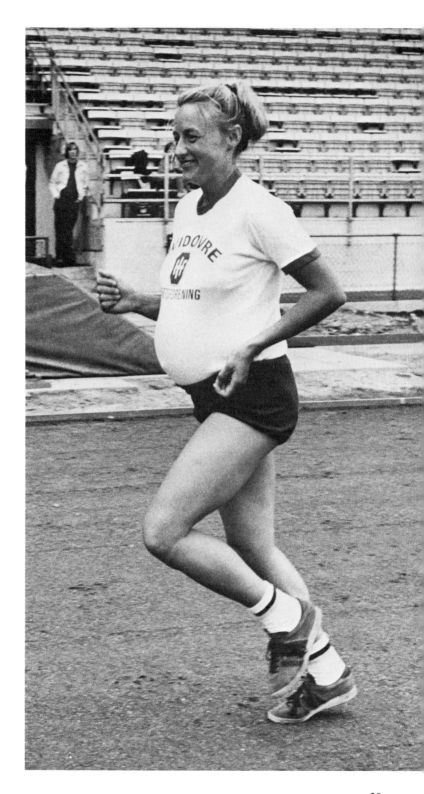

*From the visible signs
this lady's training
and fitness are within
a few weeks of
being put to the test.*

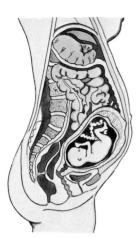

20 weeks

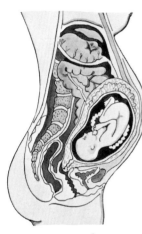

30 weeks

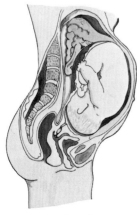

36 weeks

larger and the circular patch around them, the areola, darkens and may swell slightly.

So-called 'morning sickness' is another common early sign of pregnancy; but it certainly does not occur only in the morning. The cause of the nausea, which is usually mild, is not known. But it may be related to the large increase in circulating sex hormones that occur early in pregnancy. There may also be psychological elements involved. (This is discussed further in Chapter 8.) If nausea and/or vomiting does occur (and it seems to in about 50 per cent of pregnancies), it starts about the sixth week of pregnancy. It has nearly always disappeared by the 12th week and often by the eighth.

The pregnant woman may find that in the early weeks she urinates more frequently than usual. The kidneys work overtime early in pregnancy, probably again as a result of the increase in sex hormones, so that the bladder fills more quickly than usual.

The later signs of pregnancy become obvious as the fetus and the uterus grow in size. Estimating the height of the top of the uterus in its position beneath the abdominal wall is an age-old method of estimating the stage of pregnancy. It is not always accurate because some pregnant women have, for example, either fat or very thin abdominal walls and this can confuse the estimation, but it is helpful for general assessment.

At about 20 weeks of pregnancy, the top of the uterus has reached the level of the mother's umbilicus or navel. This is regarded as a rough midpoint in pregnancy.

Until 20 weeks, the uterus top rises the breadth of two fingers above the front of the pelvic bone every two weeks of pregnancy, having appeared above this bone at about ten weeks.

After 20 weeks the uterus top rises the breadth of two fingers every four weeks until it has reached the front centre of the rib-cage at 36 weeks.

Towards the end of pregnancy, the fetal head is pressed downward and engages in the birth canal entrance of the pelvis. This means that the top of the uterus is lowered and at 40 weeks (term) it will be where it was at about 30–32 weeks.

The small splits in the skin layers that sometimes appear in pregnancy are caused by the stretching of the abdominal wall and are not serious. They are called stretch marks or striae and are pale reddish. They fade into a whitish colour after pregnancy.

Around the 18th to 20th week in first pregnancies and the 16th to 18th week in later pregnancies the first fetal movements may be felt. They are initially very slight and seem like a tremor. This 'quickening' (as in 'the quick and the dead') signifies life. It used to be thought that these early movements reflected the first life of the fetus.

These movements become much stronger as pregnancy proceeds. The developing fetal limbs push against the uterine wall and can be seen and felt through the abdominal wall.

Fetuses have quiet periods (perhaps actual sleep periods), and these vary in length and degree of activity. These phases are often not synchronised with maternal rest or sleep periods, and thus, while normal and good signs, can be disturbing to the mother. The pregnant woman can become anxious when the fetus is quiet for a day or more after being notably active. This prolonged fetal rest, is, in fact, quite common and does not signify anything amiss unless it lasts for more than a day. However, if the condition persists for longer than a day or so, medical opinion must be sought.

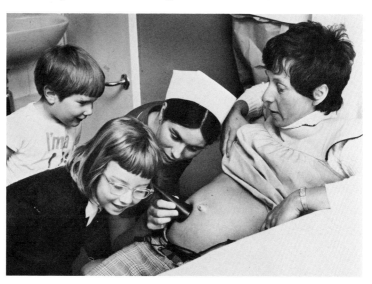

'He says what number did I dial? ...'

Obstetricians listen to the fetal heart sounds, their rate and regularity, for many reasons. These sounds not only confirm that the fetus is living, but are also a good monitor of its health, especially as labour nears. Fetal heart sounds can usually be heard from the 12th week and are almost always detectable after the 16th week.

Changes in feelings and functions

A fertilised cell needs vast amounts of nutrients and oxygen in order to multiply, then grow and develop into a human infant in 40 weeks. The resultant waste products have to be removed. The mother's blood supply bathes her side of the placenta's cells, where oxygen, nutrients, trace elements and other substances are given by the mother and taken by the fetus. The placenta conveys these substances to the fetus's own circulation.

Early in the pregnancy large quantities of the sex hormones oestrogen and progesterone are produced by the placenta cells. These help adjust the mother's metabolism and function to the demands of the fetus. Early in pregnancy there is little problem for the mother in supplying the embryo and fetus with its requirements of nutrients and oxygen.

But later the demands on the mother's energy production increase considerably. By late pregnancy the amount of the mother's blood, which is the main vehicle for transport and collection of oxygen and substances, is increased by about 1 kg (2·2 lb). This means that the heart must work harder than usual, pumping in greater volume at a faster rate.

The basic nutrients a mother produces for her fetus are good for her own metabolism and function too. This could create difficulties: she could use them up herself, for example. Moreover, the nutrients need to remain in her bloodstream for longer than usual in order to be constantly available for her fetus. Nature solves this problem in an ingenious way. The healthy pregnant woman generally leads a slower life: she conserves energy by slowing down, both physically and mentally. She lays down fat stores, by not using up her full energy intake. This is another source of energy for her fetus.

This slowing down seems to be a result of the presence of one of the group of hormones that circulate in much-increased amounts during pregnancy. This is an advantage to mother and fetus. Of course, it can worry a particularly active and bright woman—especially in her first pregnancy. She should accept the change without concern: she will 'recover' within a few weeks of the birth.

It seems that the fetus usually has first call on the mother for its basic needs, psychological as well as physical. Cases of severe maternal malnutrition illustrate the fetal 'first call'. Fetal growth and development is certainly affected, but remarkably little: the infant may well be born within normal limits of size and function. Nature has clearly organised for the benefit of the fetus a system involving the psychological, physiological and behavioural priorities of the mother-to-be.

Antenatal care

It's definite. Pregnancy is a fact. The doctor has confirmed it. But who is 'the doctor'?

A family doctor who knows the background and medical history of the woman concerned is well suited to look after health and other matters during pregnancy. This can be good for both sides. In Britain and on the continent of Europe the mother-to-be may also be attended by a midwife, with whom she builds a continuous relationship up to, during and immediately after the birth.

On the other hand, it may be more practical or desirable to attend a regular antenatal clinic which has all the expertise, tests, and so on for regular examinations. Here 'the doctor' may, in fact, be a team.

An obstetrician—a specialist? Very desirable for the birth, when the family doctor is inexperienced and unskilled in this area. Some pregnant women are more comfortable and confident

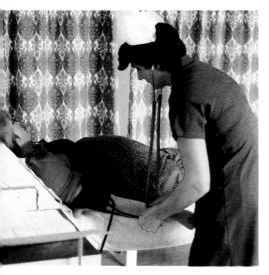

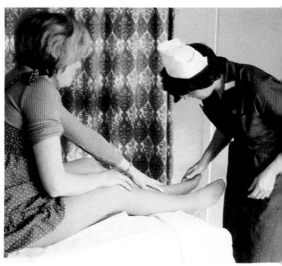

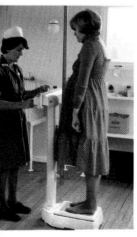

Regular medical checks, weekly near the birth, are vital: any trouble is best spotted early.

if they are under the care of an obstetrician throughout their pregnancy. In a normal pregnancy such specialised care is not specifically necessary: however, nervousness is understandable, and it is simple to ask the family doctor for a referral right from the start.

It is vital that a pregnant woman has regular medical examinations. This is good antenatal care, whatever her choice of 'doctor'. If trouble is spotted early, there is more chance of its being dealt with successfully.

The best time to start antenatal care is when the second missed menstrual period would have happened. At the first visit, a woman will have her past health story taken; and a complete medical examination will determine her general health. Important 'base-lines' will be determined, including body weight, abdominal size, blood pressure and breast size. At subsequent visits, the physician will see if things are progressing normally and whether changes from these base-lines are acceptable or not. Ideally, visits should be every four weeks up to 28 weeks of pregnancy, then every two weeks until 36 weeks, and finally weekly.

Pregnancy as a condition

It was not very long ago that a woman was labelled as being in a 'delicate condition' during pregnancy. She was therefore treated that way, and everyone fussed over her. So-called 'demanding' activities were barred to her. For her, it was 'proper' to stay at home, to rest, read, get plenty of sleep, and knit or sew.

It cannot be stressed enough that pregnancy is *not an abnormal condition*. It is a vital part of human existence. Today it is acknowledged that there is precious little a healthy pregnant woman cannot do. This includes exercise, sport, and her regular job. Of course she should avoid getting too tired. But busy, employed women are often much more relaxed and happy if they continue to work during pregnancy. In some countries maternity leave must be given, if needed, in the last weeks of pregnancy. In any case it may be sensible to arrange a shorter working day.

A word or two on the psychological influence on the fetus. First, a fetus is completely embryologically formed by about the eighth week of the pregnancy. Thus, no acute mental crises, shocks, or stresses in pregnancy can be associated with congenital malformations, serious or slight, being found in an infant at birth. It is worth emphasising this, for there is an extensive folklore on this subject, and the handing down of traditional misinformation can cause much distress.

Secondly, the only specific way a fetus is 'connected' to the mother is by blood supply. The placenta cells transport many different substances across the placenta which eventually finish up in the fetal circulation. But there are no connections between the maternal central nervous system and that of the fetus.

Nevertheless, studies have shown that the fetus can be affected by the mother's psychological state. The maternal–fetal blood circulation conveys hormones and oxygen, as well as nutrients; and these may affect the fetus if a mother is psychologically upset.

Studies have suggested a relationship between psychological stress in the mother and below-average development of the infant's ability to move at birth; between anxiety and fatigue during pregnancy, and restlessness, crying and vomiting in the young baby; between anxiety in pregnancy and an increase in crying of newborn infants. These and other studies have claimed to show pre-natal and/or genetic psychological influences on fetal growth and development.

The whole area is fraught with research difficulties; up to now there is a lack of hard evidence from good studies to disentangle genetic from pre-natal psychological influences. So we need to be cautious about accepting the possibility that a maternal psychological factor can alter the behaviour and psychological status of her fetus.

Exercise in pregnancy

The uterus is a muscular thick-walled container that gets bigger and bigger in pregnancy. It is supported within the abdominal cavity by two strong ligaments on either side—like guy ropes. The mother's abdominal (tummy or belly) wall, which is quite thick regardless of the amount of fat present, covers the abdominal cavity.

The uterus contains the amniotic fluid or 'waters' within two tough membranes or 'envelopes'. Inside this fluid compartment the fetus floats, grows and develops. In this way, protection is provided for the fetus. A pregnant woman's fall need not mean damage to the fetus. On the other hand, pregnant women should not carelessly imagine that the fetus is immune to all damage.

When labour comes, it is ideal for the woman to be in good physical shape. During the pregnancy she should continue to practise her usual exercise or sport as far as she can without strain. There is no need for the busy housewife who does not usually exercise or play a sport suddenly to go overboard and start. But if swimming is usual and enjoyed—continue swimming; similarly, riding, gardening, walking. There is no need to avoid travel during pregnancy. (Some airlines may need a certificate of 'good health' for a woman who is more than 30 weeks pregnant.)

Weight gain and diet

Different female body frames react differently to pregnancy. At one extreme, some healthy women can carry their normal-sized fetus right through to normal birth remaining virtually sylph-like and able to wear their usual clothes almost to the end. At the other extreme, some healthy women look and feel very large from very early on.

Generally pregnancy does not permanently ruin the appearance. Only if a woman puts on excessive weight and lacks exercise will pregnancy seriously affect her figure.

Obviously all pregnancies result in weight gain. Some of this is accounted for by the growing fetus, the placenta and the amniotic fluid. The enlarging uterus and the breasts also increase in weight. But there are also less obvious factors. The hormones which increase during pregnancy cause both the retention of water and the storage of fat, probably as an energy source. Also, as already mentioned, extra blood is made, and the volume of blood circulating increases.

Below is a list of the *average* percentages that each contributor makes to the total gain of a healthy pregnant woman's total body weight. The *average* normal gain of weight over the duration of a pregnancy, is about 12·5 kg (28 lb).

	Proportion of weight	Weight
Fetus, placenta, and amniotic fluid	35·2%	4·5 kg (9·9 lb)
Body water increase	32·0%	4·0 kg (9·0 lb)
Fat stored	16·0%	2·0 kg (4·5 lb)
Uterus and breasts	8·8%	1·1 kg (2·5 lb)
Blood volume increase	8·0%	1·0 kg (2·2 lb)
	100·0%	12·6 kg (28·1 lb)

This weight gain does not take place regularly and smoothly

over the whole 40 weeks. Up to 20 weeks it amounts to about 3·5 kg (8 lb). Then the fetus grows rapidly, fat is deposited, and the water starts to be retained. So the second 20 weeks produce an average weight gain of 9 kg (20 lb).

There are wide individual variations and all these figures are guides. Women who are overweight before pregnancy are usually advised to watch their weight carefully; and those who are underweight are encouraged to put weight on.

The weekly weight gain in the second 20 weeks is an important indicator of normality, or potential problems: 0·45 kg (1 lb) a week in those last 20 weeks is a good guide and makes the 9 kg (20 lb) sum come right. If weight gain amounted to more than 0·9 kg (2 lb) in a week, it might suggest that too much fat or body water was being accumulated.

Normally and usually, after pregnancy the figure and weight will return to what they were before. But if a very large weight gain, say 15 kg (33 lb), is allowed, then it can be a real problem to lose that excess.

The diet itself

The pregnant woman must see that she eats sufficient nutrients and provides sufficient energy for the growth of her fetus and for her own needs. Clichés such as 'eating for two' do *not* apply. A normal, healthy pregnant woman does not have to bother with a special diet. In general, provided that it is within a usual and normal range, the diet has very little influence on the pregnancy or birth, or on the size or survival of the newborn baby.

However, pregnant women may need an extra protein component and iron-containing foods in the diet. In some countries health services provide mineral and vitamin pills, as precautionary supplements.

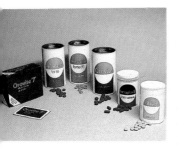

Iron supplements, vitamins and extra proteins may be prescribed or provided as a routine matter.

Day-to-day hygiene and care

Clothes

Without spending extravagant sums on special 'maternity clothes', it is possible and often desirable for a pregnant woman to dress attractively and feel attractive. Comfort is important to her physical well-being. Constricting elastic below the waist is to be avoided as it very often tends to restrict blood flow, causing varicose veins. The breasts are enlarging and need adequate support.

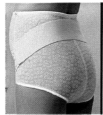
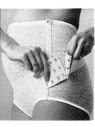
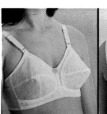
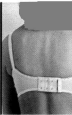

There is no reason why a pregnant woman should not look attractive and feel comfortable.

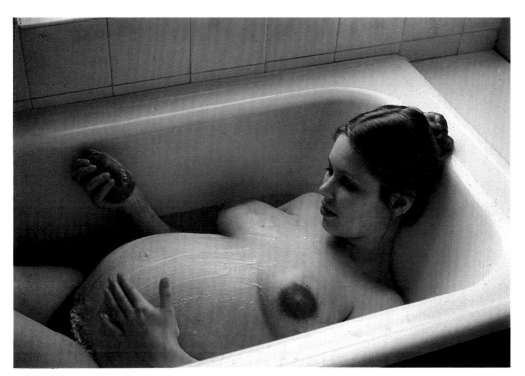

Baths

Long, soothing, warm baths are perfectly safe, and so is ordinary swimming. During the last four weeks, however, in rare cases the doctor may advise a woman to take showers and not lie in water that *could* enter the genital tract.

Breasts

The antenatal team should advise and instruct on daily breast care. The nipples need to be gently drawn out and stroked for a short time daily. And after about 30 weeks, the pregnant woman needs to be shown how to press the body of each breast towards the nipple. This is called 'expressing', and can help the milk to flow when it first comes in.

Dental care

If the natural drinking water supply is low on fluoride, a doctor is likely to prescribe a daily fluoride tablet to help the baby's teeth develop strongly, and so prevent decay in late fetal life and early infancy.

Immunisations

There is no reason why a pregnant woman should not have any necessary immunisations or 'boosters' during early pregnancy— *except* when the inoculation is with a live virus, as in smallpox or German measles (rubella) inoculations. In these cases the virus from the inoculation can reach the fetus and could cause malformation. Rubella is especially dangerous. Careful discussion with the doctor is therefore always necessary.

4　Adapting to pregnancy

One of the easiest first steps in adapting to pregnancy and the coming baby is to start acting out the role. In the early stages, when pregnancy is no more than a 'fact' and a long way from being an experience, this is the way that many women chose to practise. For practice is what is needed. Every action that raises the consciousness and increases the awareness of the coming baby will help to make him more real. As the baby becomes more real, so motherhood becomes more real, and the woman becomes more ready for birth and the immense changes that follow.[1]

Learning from mother

Many of these early practice actions are direct copies from the woman's mother, an older sister or some other model. It is here that many women experience their first difficulty, if they do not know well another woman who has had a baby. In our mobile society mothers are all too often not at hand—within easy reach, within a few minutes' walk or drive. Even though the 'official' philosophy about being pregnant and bringing up children has changed so much, and even though hospital practices have changed, a woman's own mother is still her best source of support.

In point of fact, a woman's memories about what her own mother did provide no more than a starting point for her learning. As every new facet of pregnancy and motherhood comes up for examination, her mother is the first person to whom the woman naturally turns. But having obtained her ground or reference point there, in almost all cases a woman will move on to seek her models in women of her own age. It seems that a woman must keep her mother as her mother, and not let her become an equal. Some mothers will press their concern and advice too strongly on their pregnant daughters. The daughters feel this as a great oppression, for a number of reasons.

A mother is too powerful. She does not permit the flexibility that is needed for a woman to find her own way through the different paths open to her. Psychologically she is too strong: her

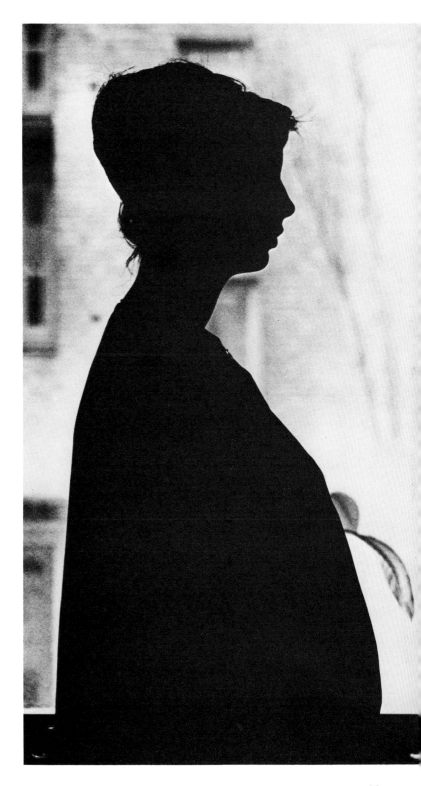

Pregnancy requires
the mother-to-be
to see herself
in a new light.

authority is too great, and she may not leave room for the process of growth and adaptation that we have described. While a mother-to-be is normally highly dependent, her mother is not the person on whom she typically chooses to depend. The mother's influence would be to keep her daughter too much in her own child state, and so disturb that ambivalence of dependency and growth that helps a pregnant woman to prepare for her new status as mother and parent.

None the less, mother remains one of the two most important single figures (the other being the husband) in most women's pregnancies, particularly in their first. It is often the case that a mother-to-be who lives at a distance from her own mother will make sure that one or other of them makes at least one special trip during the nine months, so that she can 'touch base' before moving on. In this relationship it is very important that a woman get the implicit 'permission' from her own mother to make the change from daughterhood to motherhood in her own right. If her own mother resents her growing up, a woman can feel guilty and inhibited about *daring* to assume the role of mother, having previously filled the role of daughter. If a mother feels threatened by her daughter's pregnancy, she can freeze her daughter's capacity to take responsibility for a child.

Learning from friends

Close friends can also help to provide models—especially in practical matters such as appropriate clothing, and how hard to work or how much to relax during pregnancy. Thirty years ago virtually every woman wore specially bought maternity smocks. Now a pregnant woman is just as likely to wear a loose blouse over jeans with the fronts left undone. But for the young woman pregnant for the first time, such practical questions are new and important. It is not a question of what is in fashion for pregnant mums (except for a minority, who may not be doing themselves any favours by letting such conventions sway their behaviour and mood), but of what *must* be done in the circumstances.

There may be an element of play-acting involved. 'What do *they* do, those other pregnant women? What must *I* do, to be pregnant?' If it stays at the level of acting, such moves will not help. Usually, however, they are the prelude to understanding, when the actions are incorporated into a general adaptation to change.

The drive to find out may be intense, although the questions may sound casual, the woman appears nonchalant. She should not follow every word of advice given to her, nor emulate every other pregnancy that she hears about. Apart from anything else, there will be too many contradictions, since every pregnancy is different, both biologically and psychologically. But she will be choosing which of the alternatives she feels fit her best.

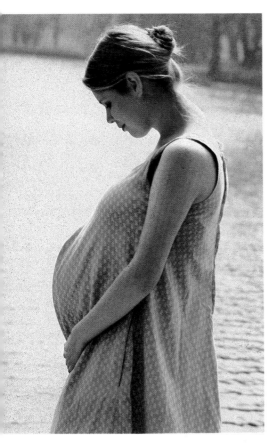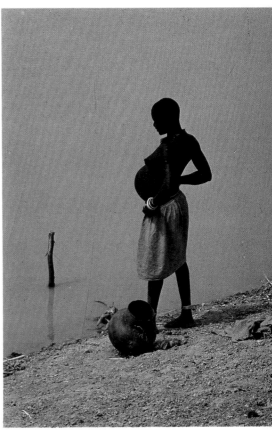

Such practical questions as what to wear, when pregnancy is the most notable thing about you, are answered according to custom and climate.

Some of the thinking that goes on in this stage is what psychologists label magical. If a woman's mother had all girls then she may imagine having all girls herself, and may well be convinced that she is bound to produce no boys. If her mother had long labours, short labours, dry labours, easy or hard labours; if her mother had all her children in the spring; then a woman may feel a strong pull to expect the same of herself. She may *know* that there is no chance of a close resemblance. But if her own conception date is two or three months too late to have her child at the same season as the one in which she and her own brothers and sisters were born, she may still feel partly convinced that her dates must be wrong and that she will fall into pattern. 'It's silly, I know,' she might say as head and heart fall out of step.

Protective folklore

Special diets are a feature of pregnancy. Books on biomedical management in pregnancy give sound advice, such as do not eat for two, do drink a lot of milk and so on. But (unfortunately) this is book-learning, and many women prefer to turn to their friends and mother for advice on what to eat and what to avoid. Many strange preferences and taboos result. The importance of these to the mother is not actually dietary. They form part of the process of being pregnant, and that process, it seems, is felt to be better learned from flesh and blood that has actually given birth to flesh and blood than from books.

Even when 'facts' are picked up from the mass media they tend to pass into a special women's folklore of pregnancy that has an existence of its own. For example, there was a much-publicised scare a few years ago that if a pregnant woman ate blighted potatoes her baby would have spina bifida. What little evidence there was then has since been discounted and there is no longer thought to be any such effect. Yet the belief survives, and is passed on from one year's pregnant woman to the next.[2] No doubt this reflects the specially defensive, self-protecting state of women in pregnancy—although there is the additional factor that since the Press concentrates, on the whole, on bad news, the clearance of potatoes never received the publicity that the first alarm did.

New friends

The intensity of the search for models and information is often reflected in an abrupt change in the woman's circle of friends and acquaintances. Suddenly she singles out for special attention those who are, or who have recently been, pregnant. She may never have noticed before how many women she knew had young children or were themselves pregnant. Even women who have tended to be solitary, content with one or two friends and the company of their husbands, may in a few weeks considerably enlarge their circle to include models and sources of information. Every opportunity may be taken of striking up friendships or at least conversations. Encounters that previously amounted to no more than an acknowledgement in the street or a word at the launderette now become opportunities for an intimate talk in which experiences are exchanged.

Friends multiply during pregnancy-especially recently-pregnant friends interested in a new member of 'the club' and anxious to pass on the rules.

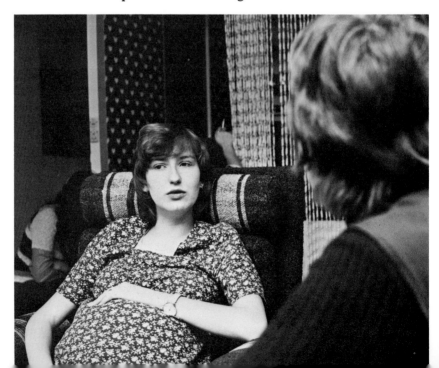

42

A kind of tunnel vision sets in, and conversations become dominated by babies. Illogically, women often feel obliged to apologise for this, as though the interest were quite illegitimate. Some women in fact do find the 'baby talk' actively distasteful; nevertheless even they may join in, or at least listen and make themselves reluctantly receptive, so powerful is the need to know. If a woman does not—if her distaste is strong enough to shut out the talk and the experience—then she may be laying up trouble for herself and her child. Reva Rubin,[3] who has studied how women adapt to pregnancy, has named this kind of behaviour in the first stage of pregnancy 'mimicry'.

Practising mothering

As pregnancy progresses and the woman learns more and adapts more, she moves into a role-playing stage. She may now seek out mothers with young babies and offer to play a part in small items of caretaking. Generally this is felt to be possible only with the children of sisters, sisters-in-law, or very close friends indeed. This is another reason why the dispersal of families has proved such a handicap to young mothers and mothers-to-be. It means a young woman's friends are likely to be those she meets at work, and even they may live some distance away. A close community which can share and teach in this way is almost a rarity.

A woman may find herself tentatively offering to change a wet nappy or diaper (a soiled one is usually felt by both sides to be too great a commitment), or simply to handle the baby. She may feel shy of asking to do something as small as holding the baby; it would be a service to her to offer to let her do so. A common move is to help to feed a toddler or to offer a rusk—or just a toy—to a smaller child. Such steps can be very reassuring for a woman who is pregnant for the first time. The experience of holding and of doing even a small mothering task can go a long way to making the unknown known, to demonstrate to the woman that she is capable of becoming a mother who gives and takes care.

Personality changes

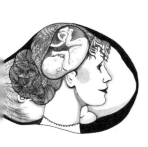

As she moves further into the pregnancy, a woman may find herself going over her past. She may find herself caught by reminiscences and daydreams of details from every stage in her life. She may recapture and relive vividly a moment in her mother's kitchen when she was little, an episode at school in the company of other girls, the mood of a family holiday, the atmosphere in the shop or office where she worked, the first meeting with her husband, an event in courtship and the wedding. These are not the random musings of an idle mind. On the contrary, they are evidence that the mind is hard at work resorting data from the past, reviewing it and reassessing it.

In every personality, echoes from the past play a large part. Large aspects of identity may derive from what a person has experienced and achieved. How a person reacts to current events and plans for the future depends to a large extent on the influence of these 'past' parts of the self. When a very large change looms in the future, then those parts of the self that survive from the past must be reviewed to see how they fit with the best future outcome. Those parts that fit are retained; those that do not fit must be discarded. Gradually the older parts of the personality are diminished in importance, and then perhaps discarded altogether.

Pregnancy seems to be one such time when the personality is reviewed. The actual changes take place in the weeks after the birth. Then, as the new self and the role of mother become established, the old self is reorganised. This is what makes the time after a birth such immensely hard psychological work.[4]

Every pregnancy takes the process of identity and personality change a little further. Early and less intimate parts go first—the schoolgirl, the worker, and aspects of childhood. The career woman, having invested more of herself in her career, will lose less of that part of herself than a woman who worked only to help the family budget until such time as she became a mother.

During the course of these changes the way the mother-to-be rehearses her pregnancy and the coming birth and baby changes. From the early external stereotype of 'how-does-one?' to which she seeks to conform, the woman increasingly moves to a more pragmatic 'how-do-I?' of 'how-shall I?'. (This stage is termed 'introjection—projection—rejection' by Reva Rubin.) As she builds up her practice and comes to know her own behaviour and attitudes a little better, the woman is able to compare herself with the models she has been using, her mother, her friends,

Practice makes perfect: it is useful for the first-time pregnant woman to learn from a friend who already has a baby—even if the 'borrowed' baby seems not to approve (below).

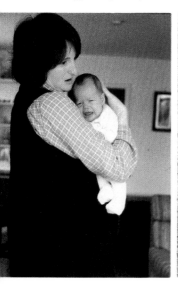

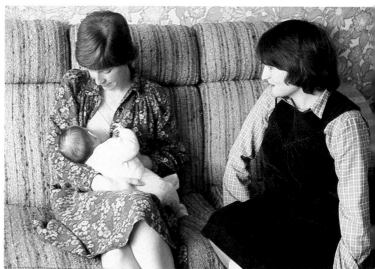

public figures or 'ideals' in books. She will be able to recognise what patterns of behaviour and what feelings match her own. On the basis of such comparisons she will be able to recognise those areas in which she feels she is doing well, and those in which perhaps she still has work to do. Models are rejected or accepted more critically as the woman grows more familiar with and sure of her own psychological and biological processes.

The mother-to-be will find that her conversations with friends change as time goes on. As she becomes more familiar with the business of being pregnant, she is able to ask questions that lead her towards some particular piece of information, to confirm or discount an idea or an attitude that she has worked out for herself. The sense of incomprehension and ignorance will give way to knowledge and understanding and to an awareness of what the things are that she does not yet know or comprehend.

Getting to 'know' the fetus

At three months most women find it difficult to believe that the fetus is 'really there'.[5] They never imagine the fetus or try to form a mental picture of it, and even those who accept pregnancy fully as a fact find it difficult to feel that the fetus is actually a baby human being, and a real person. But a sizeable minority—about a third—have already taken that step. They already believe that the fetus is a real person. They talk about the baby with affection and concern, and are aware of the close biological interaction between the two of them.

The fetus: once visualised, its 'personhood' is established.

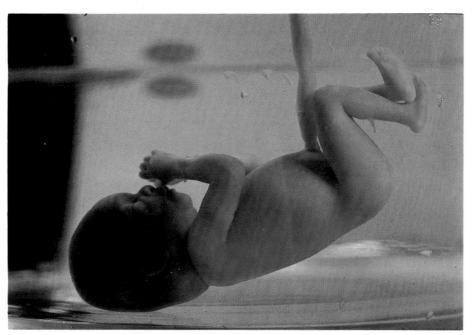

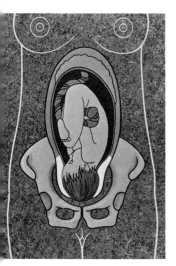

What all the mental preparation has been about: the beginning of the end of a uniquely intimate relationship.

The women who feel doubt and uncertainty about the status of the fetus are usually more pleased than not with their pregnancy, and many are thoroughly delighted. The reason that they find it hard to relate to the coming baby may well be that they have a good deal of psychological work to do in themselves in adapting to the coming child and motherhood. The fact of pregnancy is certainly enough for them to absorb for the time being.

By five months most women have felt the 'quickening'—the baby's first moves detectable by the mother. It was formerly thought that this was the point at which the baby started to move, and in a manner of speaking ceased to be merely a fetus and became an unborn baby. Now we know that the fetus moves gently, rhythmically and steadily and would react to being touched, if that were possible in his normal environment, from as early as six or seven weeks of gestation.

The quickening is thought to be a most important event in the course of pregnancy, for it is the point at which the baby makes his presence both definite and known to the mother by his own actions. His movements become increasingly strong and vigorous, and for the next few weeks he will be tumbling and turning in the womb, now this way up, now that. There is no set pattern as to which way he turns. During the last few weeks he becomes so large that the walls seem to close in upon him and make very cramped quarters.

At five months most women are able to respond to the baby as a real person. He is no longer 'it', or 'the thing' or some other depersonalised name, but 'the baby'. Many couples avoid choosing a name until the birth, and in the meantime give the baby a nickname that will serve him until birth. Sometimes this is due to the obvious uncertainty about whether the baby will be a boy or a girl. Some couples overcome this by choosing two alternatives, but others find if difficult to make a commitment in advance of actually seeing the baby.

As the time of birth draws near—by the 36th or the 38th week of gestation—the vast majority of women have accepted the baby as a real person. Those who earlier said that they would not be able to see the fetus as a real person until it had been born, or until they had seen it respond like a human being to themselves or another person, have almost all changed their minds.

They have not fully caught up, however. Those women who recognise the personhood of the fetus early are more likely to 'talk' to the baby. They feel that they have known him for a long time, and are already well acquainted. It is a strange sort of acquaintance, of course, for the communication is very limited. It is almost like having a pen friend who has never sent you a picture, and who writes only very short letters.

It is much easier for women to come to terms with the impending baby if they have had close contact with children before. Women from large families, nurses and schoolteachers tend to form their attachments early and strongly.[6]

Second pregnancies

Towards the end of their first pregnancy or just after the birth many women feel that they do not want to have another child. Within a few months, however, this feeling passes in the great majority of women; and they, with all the rest, have their second two or three years later. Then, as the new pregnancy begins, they may say 'What have I done? Can I have forgotten that I swore "never again"?'

Second-time mothers also have a major task of adjustment. Many women, having established a working relationship with one child (a relationship in which the husband is usually but not always involved), find it hard to imagine sharing or expanding this relationship. To have more children—to expand her conception of motherhood—the woman needs again to widen her psychological world and change her idea of the family. Even mothers with a good understanding of what is in store for them with the coming of the second child usually need to practise being the mother of two in the same way that they once needed to practise being a mother of one.

Even for mothers the first childbearing is not a complete guide to the second: fathers may find adjustment to a bigger family is hard.

These mothers will not only go over the ground they had previously covered but forgotten or set aside; they will seek out other mothers with two or more children. Now the conversations are about 'your second'; they explore the expansion of the family and the differences between children and between babies. This too is important, for the great differences in temperament between one baby and another can take mothers by surprise if they do not prepare themselves for the possibility.

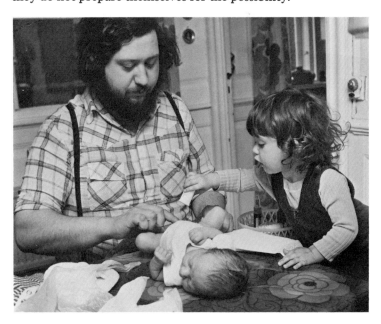

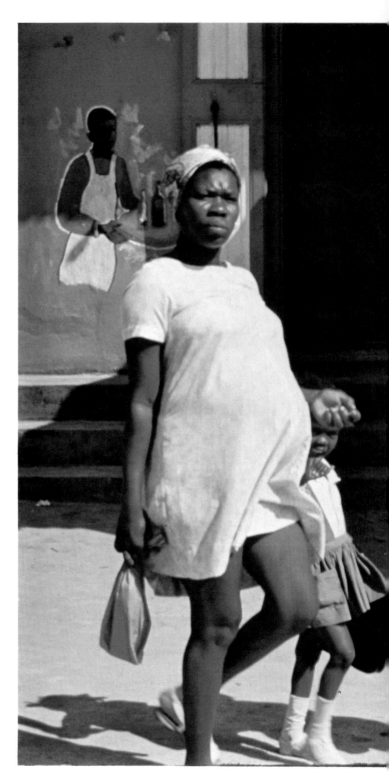

*Women are supposed
to be radiantly healthy
and happy in pregnancy—
so the myth goes:
anxiety and distress
are in fact equally
typical at this time.*

48

5 Emotions in pregnancy

The modern image of a pregnant woman is of a person in the pink of health, radiantly happy and confident, serenely passing her nine months until something we do not talk about in public happens to her and she comes home again with a nice little bundle of joy.[1]

That is the public image, to which men and women subscribe when called upon to maintain social conventions and keep up their masks of conformity in what Irving Goffman calls 'face work'. This kind of image is what sociologists call an 'ikon', a stylised representation which bears some resemblance to the truth but which is distorted in an idealised way. A real ikon is a religious object; and society's ikons, like that of the pregnant woman or the forever-feminine creature we discussed earlier, also have magical elements. Secretly we worship pregnancy and birth, both because each of us is the product of the process and because it represents the future of our kind. But, as with all religious ideals, there is another side to the coin. The secrecy which surrounds childbearing partly reflects our lack of understanding and consequent fear of the power of women in creating new life—something which men can never match, and which, in a patriarchal society, is kept firmly in the background.

The truth of the matter is a good deal different from the ikon. Pregnancy for most women is a period of doubt, anxiety, changeable emotions and psychological hard work.

All hormones?

It is commonly believed that the mood changes in pregnancy are caused by hormonal changes. Many of the books written for pregnant mothers gives hormones as the cause of emotional changeability. On the other hand, some people dismiss the role of hormones entirely, and say that it is 'all psychological'. Let us look here at the effects hormones might have.

Two main hormones play major roles in pregnancy, progesterone and oestrogen. The responsibility for mood changes has been laid at the door of both of these, and also on the possibility that in some women the two become 'out of balance'. A third hormone, human chorionic gonadotrophin, which is manufactured by the embryo in its early stages, has caused particular interest because it rises to a peak at about week ten of the pregnancy and then drops again. It would seem to be a good candidate for the villain of the piece because its life corresponds so closely with the duration of sickness during the first three months.

The same hormones play their part in the menstrual cycle, with luteinising hormone corresponding to chorionic gonadotrophin. They have also been accused of causing premenstrual tension (PMT). Different theories of the causes of PMT have their own, often fierce, support. The difficulty is that no one theory seems to apply to all cases. PMT *seems* to be linked with oestrogen deficiency in some women, but with progesterone deficiency in others. Neither seems responsible in all women. A more recent theory has suggested that a substance named oestradiol, which is produced when oestrogen is broken down in the body, can interfere with the function of the hypothalamus, a part of the 'old brain' that is very closely tied up with our emotions and motivations.

Many therapies have been proposed and tried, and as many different therapies as theories have been found to work. It sometimes appears that it is not what is in the therapy that matters, but the simple fact of having therapy.

We are left with the fact that no physical phenomenon has yet been shown to be a definite cause of PMT—or even one of the causes.[2] None the less, it would be strange if hormonal changes had no effect at all on the rest of the functioning of a woman's body and mind.

Culture and personality
It is a remarkable fact that the proportion of women who experience PMT, and the intensity of the distress that they feel, varies from culture to culture. The psychologist Karen Paige has found marked differences in the psychological experience of menstruation among Catholics, Protestants and Jews, and she believes that these differences can be traced back to the different cultural and religious approaches to women and to the human body.[3] Yet all three groups of women obviously have the same hormonal mechanisms.

It seems probable that the hormonal changes of menstruation cause an underlying low-key change in the physical system. Some women are more aware of this than others. Humans are normally quite remarkably adaptable to their environment, both internal and external. Something extra is needed to explain why some women suffer more in response to their bodily changes, and this appears to be the influence of psychological expectations. These are formulated by the culture in which the woman lives, and shaped by her own personality and family experience.

Women who score high on the 'neuroticism' scale tend to suffer more menstrual distress than women who score low.[4] This is because they react more to underlying hormonal changes.

The responses women get from people around them interact with their individual tendencies. During the premenstrual period women are much more susceptible to 'conditioning' by others, and, also, less likely to unlearn a response they have adopted earlier.[5] This means that during the premenstrual period women are on the whole more prone to pick up whatever behaviour is expected of them. If the responses they are 'taught' at this time are neurotic, then not only will they adopt them very easily, but their increase in neuroticism will make them more prone to learn more of the same lesson in following months or years.[6]

The same thing happens to women on some kinds of oral contraceptive. The fact that such pills mimic pregnancy in some ways, and that women's neuroticism scores tend to rise during pregnancy, suggests very strongly that some women are susceptible to conditioning during pregnancy.

So although the hormonal changes during pregnancy are unlikely *in themselves* to produce changeable emotions except perhaps in a few women where the changes are very large, they do make it more likely that a woman is going to react both to the changes in her own body and to the role to which society allocates her.

The role of anxiety

Even the happiest pregnancy imposes stress, but it can be of the same exhilarating kind as mountaineers feel.

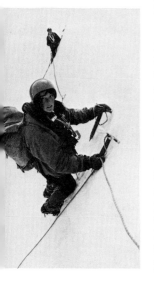

The medical profession tends to take it for granted that childbearing is a normal function of women. This being so, some doctors have tended to brush aside the feelings and anxieties of many pregnant women as irrational and irrelevant disturbances in what is a perfectly healthy process. Other doctors recognise the stress of pregnancy and are more inclined to react sympathetically to women's fears. But they still treat them as an unfortunate side effect.

Yet fear and anxiety are not only an inevitable part of pregnancy, they play an important part in preparing a woman for the last three months, for birth and motherhood. That may seem paradoxical. This is partly because it is easy to misunderstand anxiety. Anxiety and stress usually seem to us something unpleasant, perhaps even damaging, that we would be better off without. Books and articles are written on the importance of avoiding stress and how to get rid of anxiety.

For most of us, however, achievement in any form is impossible without the experience of stress and anxiety. The biologist Hans Selyé suggests that we need two words to replace the single term stress. Eustress is the word he proposes for the stress that is pleasant or constructive, like that experienced by mountain climbers or actors, and dystress the word for unpleasant stress like that caused by an accident or bereavement. In these terms, then, if a woman is happy with her pregnancy and looks forward positively to the arrival of the baby, she will experience stress, but it will be eustress. If she is unhappy with her pregnancy, or lacks a strong framework of ideas and behaviour into which she can fit the pregnancy—if she cannot entirely welcome the coming baby—then she will experience dystress.

As we have seen, our culture and our history is such that we do not make things easy for pregnant women, and so a certain measure of dystress is almost inevitable for most. Most women handle it quite adequately, with support from their husbands and families. Some need help, and for them counselling or psychotherapy is invaluable. Childbirth classes run by childbirth educators are also very helpful, expecially because they are usually arranged to allow the mothers-to-be an active role. The women are encouraged to ask questions and discuss their pregnancies. This enables them both to explore their own situation and to compare their feelings with those of the others in the class, in a strongly supporting group. In this such classes may be more help to a woman experiencing some dystress than the standard classes given in many hospitals or antenatal clinics, useful though those are. The classes given by medical institutions tend to concentrate, understandably, on the biomedical aspects of birth, and are usually straightforward teaching occasions. Since pain in labour is associated with high levels of anxiety, and good classes reduce pain, it appears that they are beneficial in helping women to cope with dystress or anxiety linked with the birth.

Anxiety levels typically rise during the first three months, and fall again during the middle three months.[7] The early anxiety can probably be attributed to the need to adapt to the pregnancy, a task which is comfortably completed in most women by the end of the third month. Anxiety rises to a new peak as birth approaches, reflecting the large changes in the woman's body, and the approach of the birth and the new baby.

Fantasies

In the last three months many women find fears and fantasies of quite dramatic and often horrific kinds intruding into their dreams and thoughts. Many women dream of accidents in which they are mutilated. One common dream or daydream is that the baby has been born and is dead or deformed. Another involves the mother's cooking, and even eating, the baby. Some women become temporarily convinced that the baby has already died within them. Most find these dreams and feelings inexplicable and distressing. They are so universal in our culture that they can be seen as quite normal; but many women do not realise this, and conclude that they are unusual, and perhaps going a little mad—or that they are very wicked.

Dreams and fantasies of this kind are common when we are under stress. They serve the function of mental rehearsal of possible outcomes that are too remote and too horrific for us to entertain in our normal thoughts. Most of us remember only a tiny proportion of all the dreams we have (up to a third of every night's sleep is spent in dreams), but when we are anxious we

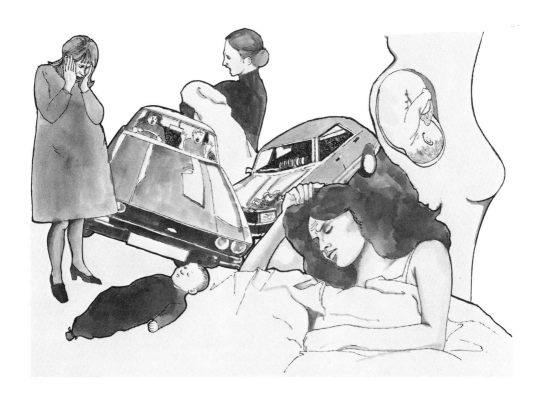

tend to sleep more lightly, and this allows the dreams to enter awareness.

It is no comfort to a woman for her husband or anyone else to tell her that the dreams are nonsense. By all means point out that the risk of having a deformed baby is small. But the psychological consequences of having a still-born or deformed child are enormous: it will help those few unfortunate couples who find themselves in this situation if they have prepared themselves even a little beforehand. What a woman with such fears needs is an opportunity to pour them out in full and discuss them with a sympathetic listener who understands the thoughts and feelings of pregnant women.

Psychological work

'I can't see that there's anything much to it. It's nature's way, and the hospital will take care of the rest.' We might envy a woman who approached childbirth with such equanimity. If we did, we would probably be wrong. Women who experience no anxiety at all during pregnancy are likely to be as badly off during and after the birth as those who experience unusually high levels.[8] It is women who experience moderate levels of anxiety who are likely to have the easiest time in labour and after the birth. The reason is that these women are doing what Irving Janis calls 'psychological work'. They are presented with a problem, a coming crisis and an encounter with the unknown— and they work at it. They learn about the kinds of things they

53

may expect and the possible outcomes. They rehearse in their minds what they are likely to experience, and they sort out which possibilities are more and which are less likely, which fears are reasonable, and which are beyond any bounds of plausibility.

Much of this work does not take place consciously. But fantasies often emerge into consciousness, and may themselves be a little frightening; often a woman does not know that she is capable of such nightmarish thoughts, and wonders what is happening to her. She may even feel a tiny bit 'possessed'.[9] Many pregnant women feel as though they are being taken over. The women who are doing the psychological work are able to handle this common fantasy, saying in effect something like, 'Of course I am being taken over—a little. That's my baby, and it's my doing, and he's going to take over a little bit of my life for quite a long time to come—I hope.'

Resolving a fantasy in this way is what marks out the psychological worker. Most women do a certain amount of psychological work of this kind during the nine months of their pregnancy. The psychologist Myra Leifer found that whatever their attitudes at the outset of pregnancy—from overjoyed to resentful—most women have moved to a more ambivalent attitude by the end of six months.

Some women will go on feeling possessed in an unpleasant way. They are not working, but worrying, and no adaptation is taking place. Their anxiety levels are high and will stay high. In birth they will be among the prime candidates for a long and difficult labour and postnatal depression.

Many women, like the one whose words we quoted at the beginning of this section, never have such fantasies. Their anxiety levels seem low, and they say they do not feel anxious. These women, too, are not working. They are denying the changes that are happening to them, and those that lie ahead. They may appear to acknowledge them, but the 'objective' knowledge they give out lacks any feeling of involvement. They may not read any literature about pregnancy and birth, claiming they know it all already. They may stay away from classes, or not pay proper attention if they go. These women, too, are among the prime candidates for a difficult labour and for post-natal depression, when the reality of their situation forces itself upon them.

When pregnancy feels like an illness

Some women treat their pregnancy as an illness.[10] They do not see it as a normal event involving normal physical changes and requiring appropriate psychological changes in themselves. Such women may be dismayed to find that their doctor does not take the same view. These women, too, are more likely to have difficult labour.

A pregnant woman who sees her pregnancy as an illness rather than as a normal biological function tends to regard herself as exempt from normal responsibilities, that is, as sick and helpless. She sees herself as having a 'condition' and she tends to be

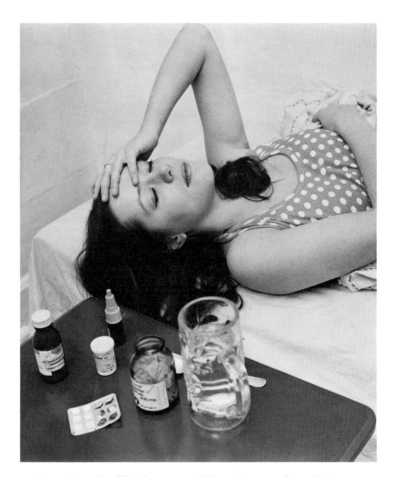

Some women see—and treat—their perfectly normal pregnancies as disabling 'illnesses'.

anxious about bodily changes and functions, as though they were evidence of some disorder. If she experiences any pain or anxiety she sees it as only natural—because of her 'condition'—and she is likely to be more subservient to and yet demanding of her doctor than other pregnant women. Most pregnant women need emotional support, especially in the last three months. These women, however, make demands on their husbands and doctors from early on.

By contrast, women who do not slip into the 'sick role' do not see pregnancy as a 'condition' ending in recovery. They tend not to worry about possible organic complications, and if they feel any pain they want to know why. When they visit their doctor it is more likely to be on an equal footing.

There seem to be quite clear differences in the social attitudes of the women with these two types of reaction. Women who accept pregnancy as normal have a positive attitude to life. They are more likely to have positive social aspirations. They want to attain, gain, accomplish or acquire things. Women who see themselves as ill tend to have negative social aspirations. Their thoughts tend towards getting away from or getting rid of

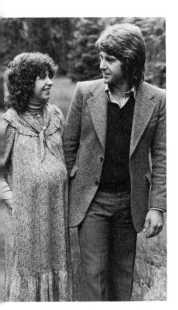

The changing personality of the pregnant woman will alter her relations with the father ...

something they see as undesirable or unpleasant, without having anything very definite as an alternative.

When we break down their aspirations into different types a further distinction appears. Women whose aspirations are for material things such as a new car or washing machine tend to be those who see themselves as ill, while those whose aspirations are for a different way of life, for a better neighbourhood, friendlier neighbours, better schools, political change and so on, tend to be the women who accept their pregnancy as normal.

Women higher up the class structure are less likely to see pregnancy as an illness. Lower-class women are more likely to experience pregnancy as an affliction. Two other factors cut across this, however. First, women with high status jobs may be more likely to see themselves as ill than those with low status jobs: for them pregnancy seems to represent a lowering of the status they have achieved through their work. Second, a woman is more likely to take the 'ill' role if her educational status is higher than her husband's. Again there seems to be a conflict between her pregnancy and the way she views her social position.

The stress caused by social mobility also leads to the feeling of being ill rather than healthily pregnant. It does not matter whether the mobility is upward or downward. If she is on the move socially in either direction, the result for her experience of pregnancy is not likely to be good.

One of the most important psychological tasks for a woman during pregnancy is to review and revise her ideas about who and what she is. Even when a woman accepts her pregnancy as biologically normal she may still feel that she is not her normal self. Dana Breen, an American psychologist who studied English women having their first babies, was amused when one of her mothers-to-be greeted her at an interview late in pregnancy with 'You haven't changed.' Breen had indeed not changed in the three months since their last meeting, but Mrs Temple had.

During pregnancy most women's self-concepts change. The change is both a result of the challenge or crisis, and their adaptation to it. It can also be in itself a cause of anxiety for some women. Much of this is to do with their earlier process of maturing. Much of the change turns on the pivot of the women's image of, and her own relationship with, her mother. A mother who controls her daughter's life very closely makes it difficult for her to make the necessary adjustments during pregnancy. A mother who is positive in the guidance she offers her daughter, but allows her room for initiative, helps her to attain the psychological adaptiveness that pregnancy requires.[11]

Dana Breen found that women who have difficulty in adjusting to pregnancy and birth tend to have a highly idealised view of what a mother should be, and they are much less likely than women who adjust well to see their own mothers as 'good mothers'. The women that Dana Breen studied who adjusted well, tended to grow towards their own mothers during their pregnancy, while those who adjusted poorly tended to grow away from their mothers in their self-concepts. Particularly interesting was how the women changed their concepts to produce this pattern. Those women who adjusted well and who saw their mothers as 'good mothers' early in the pregnancy, simply grew towards them. Those women who adjusted poorly and who saw their mothers early on as 'good', grew away from them; while if they saw their mothers as not good, they grew towards them. The women who adjusted well but saw their own mothers as not good early on, however, changed their ideas about their mothers during the pregnancy, and, so to speak, made their concept of mothers grow towards their concept of themselves.

Three into two?

'Two's company, three's none.' Every baby alters the pattern of relationships that existed in the family before it arrived. The impact of the first is the greatest, however: it breaks into the pair, the strongest of all patterns, to make a threesome, potentially one of the weakest of all patterns. Probably for this reason the effects of this challenge on the pair are felt well in advance of the actual arrival of the baby.

The question for the couple is, will the baby divide them or unite them? Both husband and wife accept the pregnancy more easily if they do not see the child as coming between them.[12] If they are highly dependent on each other, they are more likely to see the child as an interloper. Many couples marry for mutual support, and their shared activities and emotional commitments to each other leave little room for a third party, even if it is their own child. Their relationship must go through major changes in order to adapt to pregnancy and the baby.[13] On the other hand,

. . . and the birth of the baby may disrupt them or make them even closer.

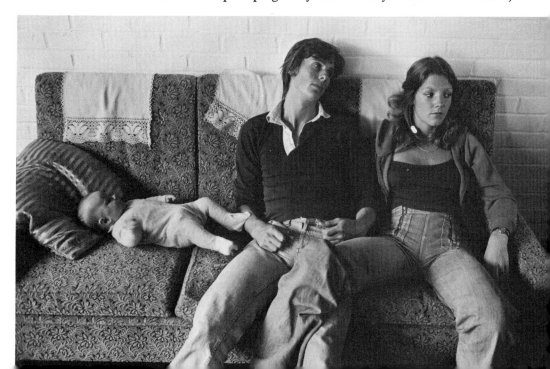

marriages in which there is a greater degree of independence between husband and wife are the ones in which the arrival of the first child is most likely to bring increased happiness and satisfaction with the marriage. In some cases this is because the relationship between husband and wife is not disturbed by the new baby, in others because the child cements a relationship that was never properly joined before.

In every marriage there is an element of negotiation over who controls the relationship. In some an agreement is made early, perhaps it is even established during courtship before the actual marriage. In others, there is a permanent jockeying for position and power. Pregnancy can have a major impact on this negotiation. A husband with a strongly patriarchal view may successfully dominate his wife as long as they are childless. But with pregnancy her own matriarchy is at least partly established, and she may recover some of the power in the relationship. Or it may be the other way round. Both partners may feel 'equal' while both have jobs; while the woman's home-based mothering may make both feel that she is now the more dependent of the two.

Esther Goshen-Gottstein compared Israeli women who had a traditional marriage in which the husband was in all things the dominant partner with women who had modern marriages in which husband and wife were on an equal footing.[14] She found that the women with traditional marriages exploited their pregnancies to gain for themselves the respect and attention of which they were normally starved.

Of course, there are large variations in how couples feel about

In some cultures the whole business of procreation, first to last, may be a shared, rewarding experience . . .

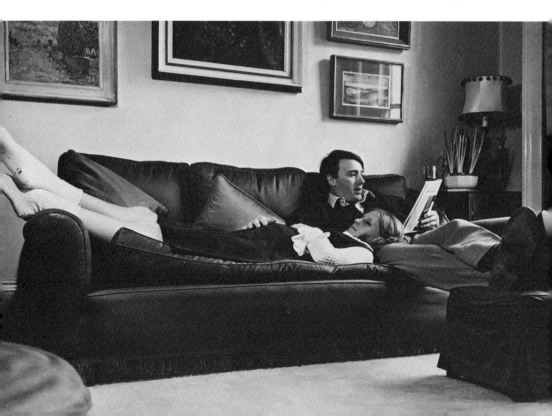

and behave towards each other during pregnancy. One might gain the impression, from neat divisions of people and marriages into types, that they remain fixed for nine months. But most career-minded men will nevertheless find themselves moved to concern over their wives occasionally, and the most devoted husbands will suddenly be overcome by feelings of impatience and estrangement from time to time. Similarly, wives who for much of the time talk over the changes they feel and their ideas about the future with their husbands will sometimes want to withdraw and be left alone for a few hours.

... and in others it is strictly 'women's work'.

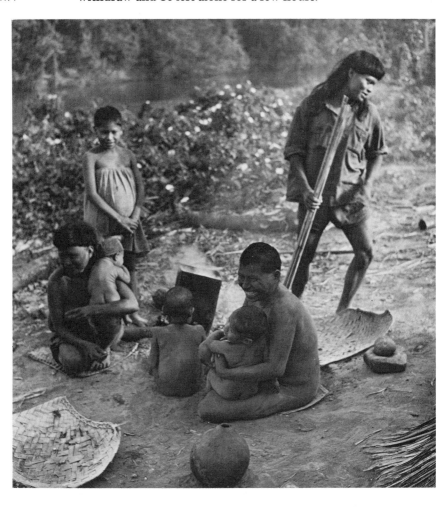

6   The body and sex in pregnancy

When we have laughed to see the sails conceive
And grow big-bellied with the wanton wind;
Which she, with pretty and with swimming gait
Following—her womb then rich with my young squire,
—Would imitate and sail upon the land.

William Shakespeare
A Midsummer-Night's Dream

Of all our biological functions giving birth is the most massive. Not surprisingly, then, how a woman views and accepts her own body and bodily functioning has an important influence on how she accepts and adapts to pregnancy.

Changes in the body

During the nine months from conception to birth the internal workings of her body force their attention on a woman as at no other time, and in a way which no man can ever experience. The change in hormones, in blood volume, in the amount of work the heart has to do, in the weight of food to be consumed and metabolised, the growing displacement of her insides, and in the last three months the pressure on her heart, lungs, liver, kidneys and other internal organs, all make their presence known in more or less direct or subtle ways. If all this were not a normal female biological event it would be intolerable.

But although the changes are normal biologically, they are not normal in the sense of being part of a woman's everyday experience. So she must do a great deal of psychological adjustment during their course. Even minor alterations in our internal body state can produce quite a substantial psychological effect. If we lose a tooth, or suffer a stomach ache, the result at the very least is likely to be distraction.

Then there is the question of the woman's external appearance. All of us who change our glasses, or who put on a hat for the first

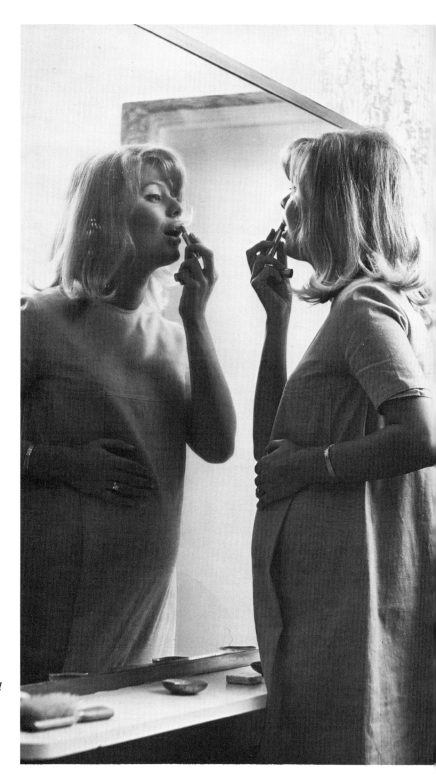

The enormous physical changes of pregnancy may make it hard for a woman to feel beautiful—but there is no reason not to try.

time, or who suffer some sort of temporary disfigurement like a boil or rash on the face, know how much our self-image and self-esteem can be affected. It may seem wrong to link pregnancy and disfigurement, but, sadly, that is how some women experience 'the bulge'. A woman who prides herself on her slimness may dislike the new expansion of her figure. A woman who already regards herself as larger than her ideal may resent a further increase in her size.

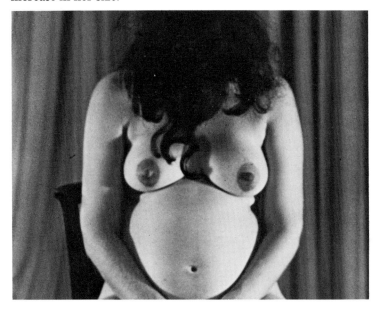

That 'a pregnant ... belly has a beauty and stateliness all its own' can be hard to accept when it is your *belly.*

Most women view the changes in their bodies during pregnancy with mixed feelings. For most there is at least some feeling of pride in the swelling of the belly, as an outward and visible sign of an inward psychological and biological change, and many women triumph wholeheartedly in their new stature. But for many the unfamiliarity of the pregnant condition, and ignorance or unsureness of how lasting the changes will be, sadly contaminate the pleasure. Many who believe as a generalisation that the weight and curve of a pregnant woman's belly has a beauty and stateliness all of its own, none the less find it difficult to be completely accepting when the belly in question is their own.

Then again, the first gentle swelling is a long way from the relatively enormous and ponderous distension of the last month. Some women who have been happy with their bulge up till then begin to make nervous jokes like 'What is it I've got in there—an elephant?' These go with the other fantasies and expressions of discomfort right at the end of the pregnancy. They are normal and no one should be upset by them.

Women who feel positively about their bodies before their pregnancy are the most likely to feel good about their changes in size throughout the nine months.

Mind and body

Women's psychology and physiology are intimately bound up with each other. During the monthly menstrual cycle a woman's whole way of thinking about herself and the world can go through quite large changes. What these changes are has been muddled up with folklore and misunderstanding. The changes vary among women. There have been many studies to try to establish effects of menstruation that are the same for all women, and virtually none of them has succeeded. The only change that seems to be consistent among all women is that during the days before menstruation, and especially during menstruation itself, most women become more anxious and have more feelings of hostility and fear. At ovulation many women are at a peak of self confidence and are open to new experiences. Therese Benedek and B. Rubenstein found that women are emotionally more passive and receptive at ovulation. They thought that this psychological state made women ready to receive the penis and sperm of their husbands and to accept any consequent pregnancy.

However it is difficult to relate what women do to what they think and feel, and impossible to be sure whether changes in behaviour are caused by alterations in physical functions, as is shown by the question of sexual dreams. During menstruation women tend to dream about men other than their husbands and fathers, with clear sexual implications. At the same time their dreams often also reflect hostility to others, destructive fantasies and a fear of being mutilated. Are these dreams 'caused' by menstruation or hormonal changes? Or do they reflect a change in women's sexual behaviour? Intercourse is most frequent during ovulation and least frequent during menstruation. It may be that the increase in sex dreams reflects an increase in the sex drive caused by the lower rate of making love. On the other hand, some psychologists think that love-making rises and falls with the sex drive itself; and that there is a rise in sex drive at ovulation related to the likelihood of conception at that time.[1]

The link between menstruation and mood is even more complicated. Mood can affect menstruation, which is made irregular or prevented by anxiety and stress, notably by conflict in marriage. The effect that a woman's state of mind can have on her bodily functions is even more dramatically shown by those women who fail to conceive for psychological reasons.

Some infertility is caused by blocked fallopian tubes. This often has a physical cause, such as disease. (This cause is probably becoming more common, owing to the rise in gonorrhoea.) In many cases, however, the block is due to the muscle that surrounds the tubes being clenched. This is not a voluntary action, but an involuntary response which is, in some cases at least, bound up with a reluctance to conceive. In many cases the cure is dramatically simple, and has no direct connection with the tubes themselves. A straightforward vaginal inspection or the passing of a sound into the womb may do the trick.[2] One case described by Dr Bernard Sandler shows how potent a woman's feelings can be in controlling her body. This woman was a farmer's wife, heavily involved in running the farm. Although she said she wanted a child and went to Dr Sandler to be treated for infertility, he assessed that unconsciously she resisted pregnancy because a child would interfere with her work. When he gave her a tubal insufflation, in which gas is passed under pressure into the womb to test for blocked tubes, he found them shut tight. When he gave her a sedative and a drug to relax her internal muscles, the tubes relaxed and the gas passed through easily. But when he reported to her what was happening, her tubes at once developed an intense spasm and became blocked again.

It is this mechanism that is probably responsible for the fact that some women, after a long period of infertility, conceive very shortly after they have adopted a child.

Sex in pregnancy

Several recent studies have shown that many women are not consciously aware of what their bodies are doing. Julia Heiman[3] wanted to find out whether women are as responsive to erotic material as men are. She found that on the whole they are, but that many of them do not realise it. There is little mistaking the outward and visible signs of male sexual arousal, of course, but self-detection is a more difficult task for women. The increased pulse, erect nipples and labia and increased engorgement of the vagina simply do not consciously register on many women.

Apart from the comparative subtleties of women's bodies, there is the strong pressure of the social convention that nice women simply do not know, or want to know, what goes on inside them. Their situation is rather like that described in the song 'I Can't Tell a Waltz from a Tango', in which a woman complains 'I don't know what my feet are going to do', although it is obvious that it is not her feet that she is really singing about. The song mocks our cultural attitudes.

In one experiment Judith Bardwick and Samuel Behrman[4] found that some highly anxious women expelled a balloon filled with water, which had been inserted into the womb, when they were shown arousing sexual material—without knowing what they had done. The likelihood of the balloon's being expelled is increased if the women is not just generally anxious but anxious about sex. Afterwards, these women felt depressed and angry. That is, these women's insides made a strongly rejecting response to sex, leaving them very unhappy. Neurotic women are sexually much less responsive, while the women who are most aware of their own sexual arousal are those who are aroused most, who respond most psychologically to erotic material, and who make love most often.

Sexuality and birth

The physical responses of a woman's body during labour and birth are very similar to those in a sexual orgasm. Some women actually experience something like an orgasm while they are giving birth, and it may be that more women would do so if they were aware of the possibility and openly responsive to the events taking place inside them. The resemblance of birth and sexual orgasm is striking when considered in full. In both breathing becomes deep and forced, but the breath is often held. The woman may grunt and gasp, and her face takes on an intense 'drowned' look, which may be mistaken for strain and pain, but which in fact is quite different. The womb undergoes regular

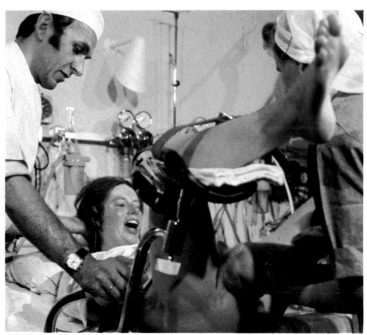

'... a return to full awareness with a feeling of rapture and joy' after the orgasm-like oblivion of the birth climax.

contractions, and the mucus plug in the cervix loosens. The whole body may move rhythmically and with a strength not otherwise achieved by the woman. During both there is an increase in sensitivity and alertness at first, and then a decline to almost complete oblivion as the climax approaches, followed by a sudden return to full awareness with a feeling of rapture and joy. The same hormone, oxytocin, plays an important part in both (although it does not naturally *cause* birth).

So it is not very surprising that the better sexually adjusted a woman is the better her experience of pregnancy and birth are likely to be. The important factor seems to be the woman's attitude to her own body and sexuality rather than her sexual relationship with her husband or other men. Women who have trouble in adjusting to and accepting menstruation at puberty are more likely to find pregnancy stressful and to experience difficulty in giving birth, with longer labours and perhaps more pain. And women who have achieved orgasm in love-making before their pregnancy are more likely to have an easier time in labour.[5] They tend to have a shorter second stage and their babies are consequently less likely to be born with the aid of forceps or by caesarian section.

One of the factors that affects a woman's sexuality is her relationship during childhood with her parents. Prudery and the repression of sex awareness in the home may discourage a girl's sexuality, but her psychological relationship with her parents is even more important.[6] Younger sisters are likely to have some difficulty in adjusting sexually, suggesting that in some families there is only limited psychological room for young girls to develop fully into females. It is not the imparting of the technical knowledge of sex that counts, but 'giving her permission' to be a fully functioning female. This is almost certainly the secret of the mysterious cures of psychogenic infertility. The examination or other procedures undertaken by a male gynaecologist serve to acknowledge to the woman her femaleness, validating her existence as a person in her own right and separate from her family, and giving her permission, or allowing her to give herself permission, to become a mother herself.

Making love in pregnancy

With few exceptions, there is no reason why a couple who want to make love during pregnancy should not do so. It is true that making love can cause contractions in the womb. These may be a temporary exaggeration of the regular small contractions that the womb undergoes throughout life, or they may be due to the hormones contained in the semen. In any case, they are insignificant compared with the contractions of labour. Only where there is already a high risk of a miscarriage should a woman abstain from sex. It is sometimes said that love-making when birth is very near can bring on labour, but at least one study has shown no evidence of this.

However, many women simply do not want to make love during pregnancy. Although it is not common for interest in sex to be lost as soon as pregnancy begins, it does happen. There is a wide variation in the amount of interest pregnant women feel in sex, and how it changes during the course of the pregnancy. Some women, perhaps a quarter, feel an increased interest which lasts until the seventh month. In about 13 per cent, the increased interest lasts right through into the last month. These women find that they make love more often and have more frequent and more intense orgasms. They are more likely to give birth easily than women who give up sexual intercourse during pregnancy.[7]

About a quarter feel less interest from the beginning, rising to three-quarters in the ninth month. Overall, however, there is a steady reduction in sex interest throughout pregnancy. Masters and Johnson[8] found a greater decrease in sex interest in women expecting their first child than in women who were already mothers: others have not found any difference. The change appears to be in basic sex drive rather than in any physical problems over intercourse. Many experience a decline in sexual activity in all its forms. There is less masturbation and less oral sex during pregnancy. Nevertheless, there is seldom a complete extinction of all sexuality. Rather there is a change in emphasis. During the course of pregnancy, many women grow to appreciate vaginal stimulation less and clitoral stimulation more.

Husbands and sex

No one seems to have studied the sex lives of husbands during their wives' pregnancy. From our own work it seems that much depends on the husband's previous attitude to his wife. Most women retain an interest and pleasure in sex when they are pregnant even when they do not feel the need to reach orgasm. It is up to the husband to reach new ways of loving with his wife. The challenge of pregnancy for a man—in sexual as in other aspects of their married lives—is to accept that his wife is changing, to find out what those changes are, and to adapt to them. The ability both to ask and to refuse is an important ingredient of sexual happiness, and never more so than during pregnancy and immediately afterwards. Many men will be pleasantly surprised at the responsiveness of their wives to their needs if they can only find the right way of expressing themselves and reaching out for help.[9]

During the course of pregnancy an expectant father must adjust to the coming baby and to the changes its arrival portends in himself and his wife. One of the strongest of all taboos in human society is that against incest, and the rarest of all types of incest is that between mother and son. Many sexual difficulties experienced by men in Western society may have their roots in this area. The exclusiveness of the nuclear family means that quite often a small boy's sexuality has nowhere to go but into unformed fantasies based upon his mother. Freud drew a very large red herring across this particular psychological trail by suggesting that it was innate and inevitable that small boys should form sexually charged relationships with their mothers.

We now know from anthropological research that the 'Oedipal relationship' is not inevitable, but is formed by the particular circumstances of mother and son, which are governed very largely by the culture in which they live.

In our culture for example some men suddenly find, when their wives become pregnant, that the girl they married is turning into a mother—a class of person with whom sexual relations are forbidden. This entails a major task of psychological reorganisation. The fact that many couples keep up love-making until late in the pregnancy suggests that either this is not a problem for them, or that it is one that they are able to cope with. But many couples give up sex when there is no biological reason to do so, and the data suggest that the husbands are at least as much responsible for this as the wives.

Many men also find that they are put off sex by the presence of the unborn child. Sometimes men have fantasies or ideas that they will damage the child, either by lying on top of it or by their thrusting. Some men feel as though they are being watched by the child. All these feelings are nonsense objectively, but they are perfectly reasonable fantasies which form part of the process of adapting to the change in the wife and to the change in the relationship from one between two persons to one between three persons.[10]

Trying new positions

Few couples need to be advised to change from the traditional 'male superior' position for love-making during pregnancy. The awkwardness for the man and the discomfort for the woman cause most couples to change spontaneously. The most favoured alternative is side by side. This position, one of the least satisfactory for men, increases during the last three months, at the expense of 'female superior' and rear entry, which are more usual up to that time.[11]

Some fathers-to-be find their partners less attractive as soon as the bulge begins to appear, others not until it is a large and inescapable protuberance. Other men, on the other hand, find

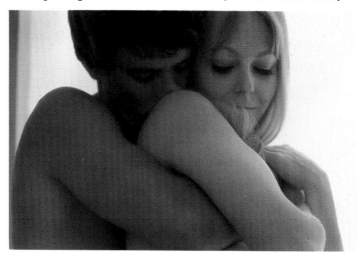

The desire just to be held may be strong during pregnancy: it is related to but not the same as sexuality.

their new-shaped partners more enticing. In the middle three months, many women go through the well known 'bloom' of pregnancy. Their skin takes on a radiant transparency, their eyes sparkle and their hair gleams. Not unnaturally, their husbands may be stirred.

The need to be held

Most of us like to be held or cuddled, especially by someone of the other sex and most of all by our spouse or sex partner. One group of medical doctors and psychologists who have made a particular study of this desire believe that it is especially strong in women.[12] Almost all women they studied reported a moderate or strong desire to be held. (There is a hint that black American women feel the desire less.) Those who denied that they wished to be held did so with such vehemence that the investigator, Marc Hollender, feels that this 'aversion' thinly covered a desire so strong that the women had to repress it.

The desire to be held is related to sexuality. Women who enjoy sex are more likely to feel the need to be held. But the two are not the same thing. Hollender believes that many women have sexual intercourse not for the sake of sex but for the sake of the cuddling involved. The desire to be held is strongly related to dependency needs. In American society, particularly, the direct expression of any form of dependency is strongly discouraged. Many of the women that Hollender interviewed found it easier to initiate a bout of love-making than they did to ask straight out 'Give me a cuddle.'

Judith Bardwick and Joan Sweben[13] also found that many women say they make love not as a response to a basic sexual drive as men do, but in order to feel close, or as a symbol of involvement, or to express love. The picture is complicated, however, because being cuddled is sexually arousing for many women.[14] The sight of a female, especially the breasts, is normally highly arousing for human males. For women, however, visual stimuli seem not to be such powerful releasers of the sex drive. They are more aroused by intimacy and body contact. It could be, then, that the need to be held is no more than a ladylike way of acknowledging the sex drive. None the less, although many women find it a useful tactic in love, there do appear to be two separate needs. In pregnancy many women tend to feel that the need to be held increases at the same time as their interest in sex decreases.

7 Fathers in pregnancy and birth

She was crying, and her colour changing from blue to pink. I held her, my bright-eyed little child, and she looked right at me and quieted in my arms.

Fein

As we have seen, the role and tasks of a pregnant woman in our modern, industrialised society are far from clear. So perhaps it is not altogether surprising that the father-to-be is also a shadowy figure. Indeed, he is so faint that he is scarcely visible at all. How has this come about?

Some writers suggest that modern society has pushed the father out. The changes in society brought about by the industrial revolution have increasingly separated the roles of the two sexes. Father has been driven out of the centre of the family network to occupy a position on the fringe, providing only the money by which the rest of the family—his 'dependants'—live. The psychoanalyst Helene Deutsch has suggested that the role of the father in birth has been taken on by the obstetrician. However, it is only in the USA that the obstetrician holds such a dominant position. In Europe, midwives still play a central role, and in many births, even in hospitals, in England and Holland obstetricians are only called in when something may be going wrong. So Deutsch's theory seems to be mistaken.

Nor can it be industrialisation, for men are excluded from birth in societies of many different economic types throughout the world. A graphic description of a father pacing the floor, wringing his hands and listening to the (to him) inexplicable and terrifying sounds coming from the bedroom upstairs can be found in Tolstoy's novel *Anna Karenina*, set in nineteenth-century pre-industrial Russia.

One reason given for the lack of involvement by fathers in pregnancy and birth is the theory that men's innate role in

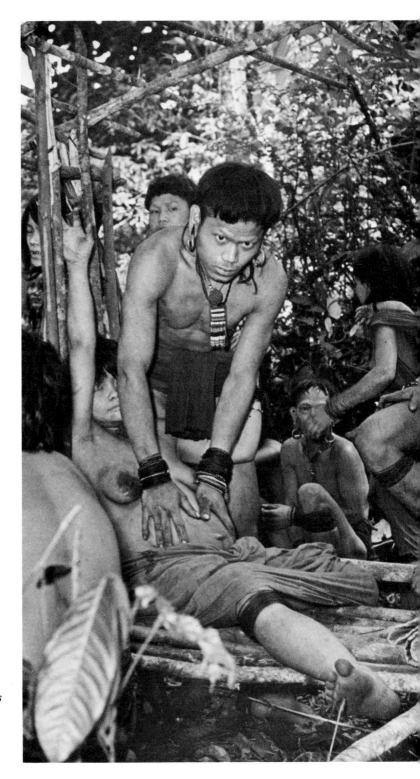

In North Borneo the whole community watches a birth—but the new baby's father has a special role in helping it to emerge.

71

reproduction ends with ejaculation. Once they have 'sown their seed', men have no further biological interest in their children. There is no good evidence for this stereotype. On the contrary, the evidence suggests that caretaking behaviour is to some degree innate in men, while perhaps not as strongly driven or well shaped as in women. It is released by the same stimuli as women's caretaking behaviour, that is, the presence and needs of young children.[1]

The impact of pregnancy

Whether they realise it or not, men are profoundly affected by their wives' pregnancies, especially the first. This impact is demonstrated by the number of men who become disturbed to a greater or lesser degree.[2] For many years this phenomenon remained a mystery. Women's symptoms could be put down to alterations in their hormones and other physical systems. But this could not explain changes in the moods and behaviour of their husbands. So the tendency was simply to ignore such changes. Only very serious disturbances were noted, and even then they were usually ascribed to something other than the wife's pregnancy.

The next step was to acknowledge that pregnancy precipitated 'mental illness' in some fathers-to-be. But what typically occurs cannot reasonably be called illness. Mood and behaviour become disturbed, changeable and perhaps erratic. These are the reactions of a person called upon to make profound psychological changes without reliable guidance, and without any support in his crisis—because nobody recognises that the crisis exists. One classic study by James Curtiss[3] of expectant fathers in the American Air Force found that few of the men and few of their doctors had any notion that changes in their feelings and behaviour might in any way be connected with their wives' being pregnant.

Such changes may include quite severe depression, or manic behaviour, even attempted suicide, robbery or burglary, and—among Curtiss's airforce personnel—insubordination and going absent without leave. These forms of behaviour are rare. More common changes include irritability, nervousness, headaches, an increase in alcohol consumption, buying sprees, or a sudden interest in a new activity outside home and work, such as a sport, hobby or extra-curricular activity.

If the stereotype of the stud who has done his job were correct, a wife's pregnancy would be nothing more than sexually triumphant for men. In fact, for many expectant fathers the contrary seems to be the case. Their sexual behaviour becomes disturbed, as though they were seeking reassurance of their own potency and prowess. The pressure seems to increase as the birth draws near. A few men attempt rape. Some exhibit themselves, or become voyeurs. Possibly the most common change is promiscuity. During the pregnancy or after the birth, the father may suddenly develop a relationship with another woman, or with a series of women.[4]

What is a father?

'What is a mum?' asked one TV advertisement. The answer that they wanted was a woman who bought the right kind of soap powder. This reflects the superficially easy definition of a mother's role: cooking, cleaning and caring for children. We know that being a mother is nothing like as simple as that; but at least it can be reduced to a simple formula.

But what is a dad? If a man takes as his answer 'someone who earns the family living and otherwise stays out of the way', he

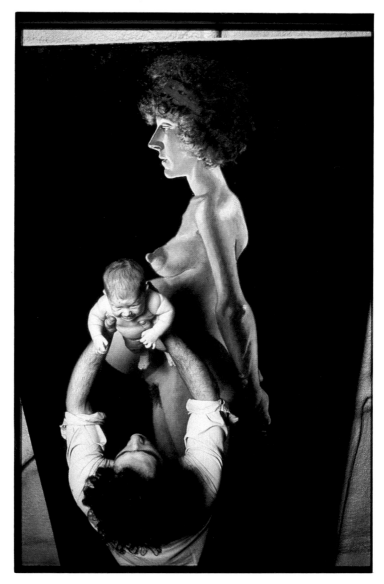

'That's what I did, and this is what I got for it ...'

may have an easy time of it. But few men take this prescription in its simplest form. They want to know what is required of them psychologically in relation to their wives and coming children. For the man who would like to take an active part in parenting his child there is very little guidance. Parenting is treated by society at large and by child-care books as synonymous with mothering.

In both the USA and the UK men have been refused social security payments to enable them to care for their children after they have been widowed or left by their wives.[5] The system apparently finds it extremely difficult to acknowledge that fathers are capable of looking after children. In Britain, on the whole, even 'poor quality' mothering is recognised as preferable to institutionalisation, but fathering is seldom seen as a viable alternative.

Fathers can be greatly helped in preparing for the baby by attending childbirth classes with their wives. It is also much easier for a father to form a relationship with the baby if he has attended the birth. In these areas progress has been made. However, the problem of parenting for men remains. Childbirth classes fill one need, but do not in themselves prepare men for fatherhood afterwards.

Studies of fathers-to-be who become seriously disturbed during pregnancy suggest that the biggest cause of their difficulties lies in the coming of the new child. Hostility and rivalry is a prevailing theme among these men: one author even described some expectant fathers' reaction to the baby as 'flight or fight'.[6] The clue appears to lie in the man's own childhood relationships with his brothers or sisters. Those men who have most difficulty in adjusting to the birth of their child are those who suffered psychologically from the birth of a brother or sister in their own childhood, leaving a trauma from which they have not recovered and which becomes reactivated by the new birth.[7]

Strictly excluded until only a score of years ago, fathers are now generally welcome in the birth chamber as comfort and support.

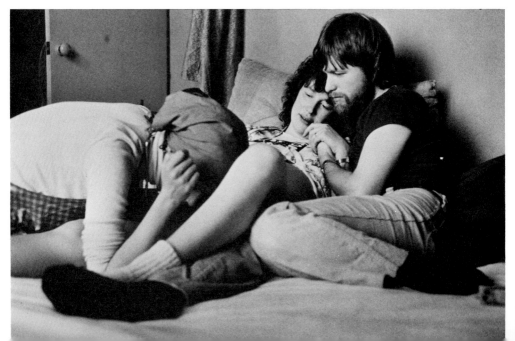

Giving support

There are good grounds for suggesting that her husband is the linchpin that ensures the smooth turning of the whole cycle of a woman's transition through pregnancy to motherhood. Several investigators have found that the husband's personality is at least as important as the wife's in determining the psychological outcome of pregnancy.[8] The more secure and emotionally supportive the husband, the more complete and successful the wife's adjustment to the changes that are required of her.[9]

The extent of the support that the husband is called on to provide naturally depends upon the wife. Some women are so well prepared for pregnancy that their husbands need provide little support. At the other extreme, some women are so unready for the transition to motherhood and so unable to cope with the burden of pregnancy itself, that the husbands are crucial to the whole outcome.[10] A woman with a moderate degree of neurosis will adjust more successfully to pregnancy if her husband is not neurotic than if her husband is also neurotic, especially if their neuroses interact.[11]

It is also easier for a woman to form a good relationship with her unborn baby when her husband takes a clear interest in the course of her pregnancy and the development of the child, and gives her emotional support throughout.[12]

Fathers and birth

The nervous father waiting in helpless ignorance in a hospital in the middle of the night has long been a standard subject for cartoonists, along with desert islands and mothers-in-law. Today, however, such men are becoming figures of the past. The time when it was suggested that there was actually something wrong with a man who wished to attend the birth of his child has gone.

Men are discovering, with their wives, that the birth of their own children can be the most joyous and ecstatic experience that this life has to offer.[13] The importance of the father's presence, however, hinges not only on pleasure or peak experiences. A father who attends childbirth classes with his wife, actively prepares for the birth and takes an active part in bringing the child into the world, generally has an easier time afterwards in adjusting to the new status of his wife as a mother, and to the presence of the new baby.

Richard Gayton has compared the experiences of two groups of fathers. One group (NCB fathers) had attended 'natural childbirth' classes with their wives and stayed with their wives throughout labour and delivery.[14] The other group (standard fathers) had not attended classes and retired to the waiting room usually at the end of the first stage of labour. Gayton found that the two groups had very different experiences.

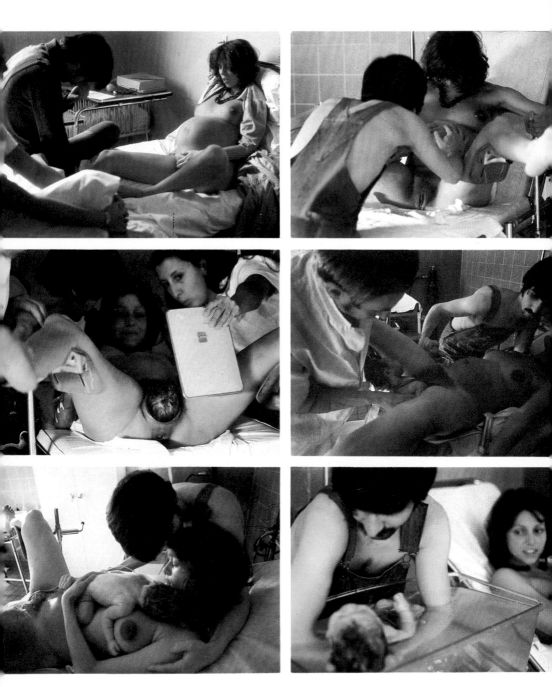

Father's birthday treat.

First, he tracked how their anxiety levels rose and fell throughout the birth process. Standard fathers were more anxious throughout the birth process until they received the news that mother and child were both well, when their feelings of anxiety dipped below those of the NCB fathers. At the beginning of labour, the anxiety level of standard fathers was substantially higher. When the wives were in hard labour, towards the end of the first stage, the anxiety of the NCB fathers rose to its highest point. Thereafter the NCB fathers became calmer, while the standard fathers, removed from the scene, continued to become more anxious, reaching a peak when they were told that birth was due at any moment.

Staying with it

The greatest causes of anxiety in the standard fathers were watching the wife in pain during labour, the appearance of the baby after the birth, a fear that the baby would be born before they reached the hospital and fears about the health of the baby. NCB fathers were most distressed if they were separated from their wives, for example, if they were asked to leave during

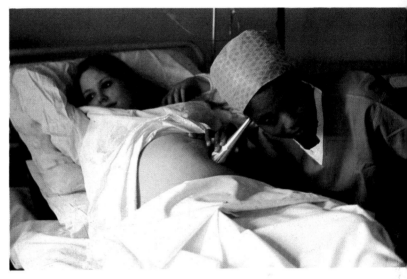

A testing time for all concerned.

'medical procedures'. The NCB fathers also found the sight of their wives in apparent pain distressing. For some this was because they felt that their classes did not prepare them adequately for the intensity of their wives' experience; in this respect their anxiety was similar to that of the standard fathers. In another respect, however, it was different, in that there was more empathy and involvement in the actual process and experience. While some of the standard fathers took flight from the situation and left their wives, none of the NCB fathers did so. Among the most distressed fathers of all were those who had expected to stay for the delivery but who were ejected by the medical staff. Only a small minority of the NCB fathers worried about getting to hospital on time, the health of the baby and the appearance of the baby, showing how their preparation had paid off.

When the baby appears

The NCB fathers who remained throughout the birth saw their babies from the moment the crown of the head first showed to

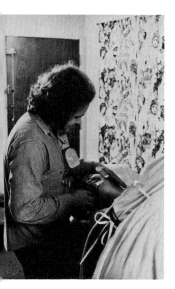

The father's presence can bring 'an atmosphere of calmness and dignity' to a time of unfamiliar stress.

the moment they appeared fully, still attached by the cord and wet, with varying amounts of blood and vernix still on them. These fathers, well informed beforehand and having seen what a baby has to endure to be born, were not upset by the baby's appearance. The standard fathers were much more likely to be disturbed.

Research on every aspect of medical treatment shows that when doctors are open with their patients, treat them in a friendly manner and give them the information that they want, the patients react positively. Birth, while not in essence a 'medical' event, usually takes place in a medical setting, especially in the USA. Here again the attitude of medical staff is important. Twice as many of the natural childbirth-trained fathers as standard fathers thought that the medical staff had been supportive and informative and had helped to allay their anxieties. In fact, the NCB fathers found much more relief from their anxieties than the standard fathers, who, apparently, felt that they were left to 'sweat it out'.

Husbands and doctors

One of the reasons that is sometimes offered for resistance by medical staff to the presence of husbands in the delivery room is that the layman might not understand all that the doctor does and 'might get the wrong idea', or even that doctors cannot afford to have their methods subjected to inspection by someone who is not necessarily 'on their side'. Richard Gayton's study shows that, on the whole, doctors have little to fear and much to gain in parental attitudes from the presence of fathers. However, there is no doubt that if 'marginal' medical practice does occur it is likely to fall under critical scrutiny. One father who watched in horror while the doctor performed what looked like a grossly exaggerated episiotomy felt that his suspicions were confirmed when the doctor remarked to a medical student who was present, 'And this is my trademark.' Such events are rare, however.

To a large extent, how a father feels about the medical staff during his wife's delivery depends upon how they treat him. If they make him welcome and permit him to play a useful and active part in the labour and delivery, he reacts favourably. If they tend to exclude him, he may react at least as negatively as those fathers left outside in the waiting room in a completely passive role.

How fathers feel

Both groups of fathers felt better about themselves after the birth, to almost equal extents. However, there were interesting differences in the nature of the changes. The NCB fathers felt that they were more adequate socially, ethically and in terms of family obligations, but their concept of their physical value had declined. For the standard fathers the changes were reversed.

In other words, the NCB fathers tended to feel that they had met a social and moral requirement that, in the present state of practice, few other men had met. They felt more united with both their wives and their children. For the standard fathers the birth of a child was on the whole a relatively simple badge of their manhood, in terms of their obligation to beget children. For the NCB fathers their close encounter with the physical and anatomical realities of labour and birth would be an influence against any such stereotyped or romantic response. Their reduced concept of their physical selves probably reflected a new realisation of the general frailty and reality of human flesh.

What fathers can do

One aspect of the father's role during labour and delivery has been likened to that of a sportsman's coach.[15] He brings his wife drinks, wipes away sweat, massages her, monitors her contractions and keeps track of her breathing and relaxation (this does *not* mean giving her orders), and gives moral support. But apart from such caretaking activity, the very presence of the father is profoundly calming and reassuring in the hospital environment, which many women find unfamiliar and hostile. Many women find that it is easier to respond to a voice they know and love than to instructions from a stranger, particularly when a change of staff may occur with a new shift in the middle of labour.

One study in Germany, in which husbands were introduced for the first time into a hospital, noted that as well as helping their wives and the medical staff, their presence 'produced an atmosphere of calmness and dignity in the delivery room.'[16]

No doubt because of this calming effect, the presence of her husband often succeeds in lowering a woman's experience of pain. There is another side to this, too. Pain is an intensely private sensation. Other people can estimate how much pain we are feeling from the expression on our faces or movements of discomfort that we make, but such cues are subtle, and it needs a good knowledge of a person before the quality of their private experience can be judged from these external signs. It is not surprising, then, that husbands are very much better at judging how much pain a woman is feeling than midwives, doctors, or even childbirth educators.

Deborah Tanzer and Richard Gayton both found that women whose husbands attended classes and were present at the birth or throughout most of the labour regarded their husbands as 'strong, competent, someone on whom in most cases the wife leaned and depended'. Wives whose husbands followed the more traditional role saw their men as 'weak, impotent and childlike, someone to be worried about rather than depended upon'. A couple in which the father remains relatively inactive in respect to the birth seems to pay a multiple penalty. Not only may his adjustment to paternity, to the child and to the change in his wife be hindered, but she is also deprived of much-needed support. She may well feel called upon to give support herself, not only to her new child but to her husband as well.

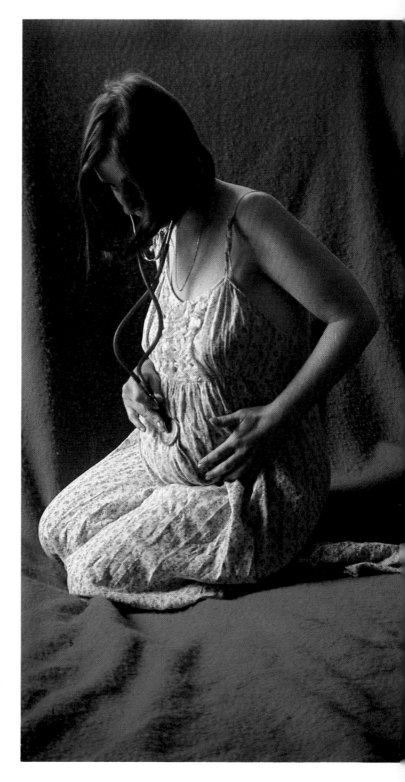

Anxiety about whether
the growing fetus
is 'alive and kicking'
is common: this is
a sensible way
to set fears at rest.

8 Problems in pregnancy

About a half of all women who become pregnant in Western countries suffer from feelings of nausea or actual vomiting, especially during the first three months. In Britain this is known as morning sickness, although it can occur at any time of day. It seems likely that many women beyond that 50 per cent have passing feelings of nausea which they never report. This phenomenon is widely believed to be a normal part of pregnancy. Many women believe it to be the crucial sign. Yet in other parts of the world the phenomenon is virtually unknown. Why is it so prevalent here?

Morning sickness

One of the new old wives' tales of the twentieth century is that pregnant women who suffer from morning sickness want to be rid of the baby. Some investigators put this theory to the test. They found that women who did not want their babies did *not*, on the whole, suffer from vomiting, while others did. The mystery remained. Why do women vomit in pregnancy? Probably the majority of women in the entire human race would be astonished at the suggestion that a normal biological process should cause anything so obviously abnormal, symptomatic of illness, not to say distressing and discomforting, as vomiting.

The clue came to the French doctor, Leon Chertok, when he noticed that two groups of women clearly did not have this problem, while others did.[1] What distinguished them? The women who did not vomit were not necessarily as lucky as one might imagine: they were France's unmarried mothers; and pregnant women seeking an abortion.

Chertok conducted psychological interviews with a number of women when they signed on for antenatal care in the third month of their pregnancies. He found that their attitudes to their coming babies could be divided quite reliably into three types. The first was a reaction of pleasure: the child was wanted and the confirmation of the pregnancy was greeted with joy. The second type of attitude was rejecting: the reaction to the pregnancy was immediate and unambiguous. The coming baby was felt to be a disaster which none the less had to be borne for various reasons—husbands, families and so on—and which the women felt had been imposed upon them by fate or by their circumstances.

Ambivalent attitudes

The third type of attitude was ambivalent. These women either felt contradictory attitudes simultaneously, or swung from one to the other. They were partly pleased and partly annoyed by the pregnancy. Even when one feeling predominated the other was never far below the surface and broke through easily.

As Chertok had predicted, the majority of the women who vomited fell into the ambivalent group. A smaller number fell into the wanting group, but hardly any were outright rejectors. Of the non-vomiters the great majority were among those who wanted their babies, with only a few among the rejectors and ambivalent group.

The idea that vomiting is a symptom of a wish to be rid of the coming baby depends upon the theory of symbolism, that psychologically one thing can stand for another. In this case the contents of the stomach have been supposed to be ejected as a symbolic substitute for the contents of the womb. Chertok's finding could be seen as a death-blow to this theory. In any case, vomiting is not uncommon in certain stressful situations, and it could be a straightforward outcome of the stress of carrying a child about which one's feelings are ambivalent and which is inexorably growing towards an event one may dread.

Here the contrast Chertok drew between unmarried women in France and in Switzerland may be instructive. At the time of his research abortion was prohibited in France but permitted in Switzerland. Unlike their French counterparts, unmarried Swiss women who became pregnant did vomit. So it seems that the woman's own desire for the child is not the only factor; her recognition of the opportunity to be rid of it also plays a part. Simple stress, then, is not the answer.

We are left with two alternative explanations. First, the availability of a termination increases the ambiguousness of the situation which causes more anxiety, and hence the tendency to nausea. Second, the opening of the option of abortion allows the woman to entertain at a higher level of consciousness her desire to be free of the coming baby. In this case if the woman rejects the opportunity that abortion provides she 'displaces' her wish to be rid of the fetus and ejects that part of the contents of her body that she has access to.

Does this mean that every woman who vomits is ambivalent about the coming baby? We must be very careful indeed about oversimplifying what is involved in this question.

There is always the possibility that hormone changes *are* responsible for at least some nausea, even though no connection has yet been reliably demonstrated. And it would be quite understandable for a woman suffering from vomiting caused by her pregnancy to feel ambivalent about her state.

No woman should fear that *because* she does not vomit she

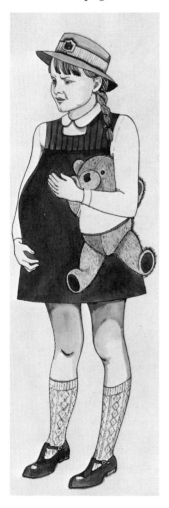

If only I was a little bit pregnant!

secretly wants to be rid of the baby. To start with, we are talking about probabilities. There are so many factors involved. A woman might feel very ambivalent about the coming baby, and yet not feel sick because other things were preventing her.

The surprise baby

There is another reason why some women may not react with nausea, vomiting or other symptoms. We said earlier that women may or may not respond consciously to the changes in themselves. Helene Deutsch has suggested that some women choose not to notice changes because they are actually denying to themselves that they are pregnant. They are not actively wanting to get rid of the baby: they are simply pretending to themselves that he does not exist. Some women in this position are those whom conception has taken by surprise. Others are those who both want and do not want to be pregnant, and in whom the not wanting triumphs for the time being. Some of these women are increasing their chances of a hard time later, both during birth and when they have the child.

Since so many women are involved, it might seem absurd to suggest that they are all ambivalent in their attitudes. When we take a look at what is involved in childbearing, however, and at the highly ambiguous attitudes that we have already described, it does not look quite so absurd. Indeed, one might almost conclude that ambivalent attitudes are the norm, and that nausea is a normal expression of our cultural approach to birth and children.

Some support for this comes from two studies, one in England and one in Sweden.

Stephen Wolkind and Eva Zajicek studied a group of London mothers-to-be.[2] They found that there was little difference in the overall attitude to pregnancy between the women who did feel sick and those who did not. There was however a difference in the way their feelings changed. The women who had no nausea started out very pleased and positive, and became rather less enthusiastic as the pregnancy went on. Those who were sick started out slightly less pleased, and developed more positive feelings during the nine months. Both groups were very much more pleased than not pleased.

The biggest difference between the groups was in their attitudes to their mothers. On the whole the ones who felt nauseous were closer to their mothers than to their fathers. They also felt that they had come closer to their husbands since they had become pregnant, while the others did not really notice any difference. The nauseous were more likely to be considering or actively planning breast-feeding, and to have given up smoking during pregnancy.

Wolkind and Zajicek feel that the differences show that the nauseous women identify themselves more with the 'culturally held' view of the female role. It may be that these women feel that sickness is expected of them, as a kind of 'badge' or public declaration of pregnancy.

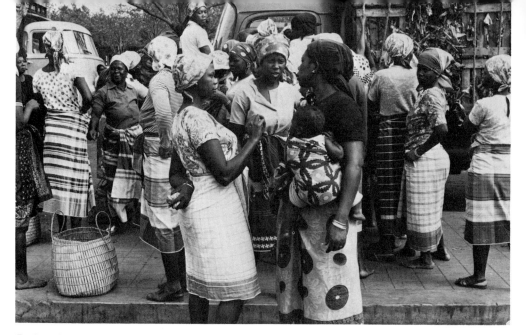

Perhaps because they accept the naturalness of maternity, African women are very unlikely to suffer from 'morning sickness' or 'toxaemia'.

The only symptom?

Nausea apart, there are very few clear physical symptoms in the first three months of pregnancy. There may be a very slight swelling of the ankles. There is usually a slight swelling of the breasts, but often this involves no more than a minor distension of the areola. Women who are at ease with their bodies and who know themselves well will have no difficulty in recognising and accepting the changes. Others will be in doubt about what is happening to them, and doubt itself is stressful. So vomiting may be the only way they have of convincing themselves and the world that they are in business and that new life, unfelt and unseen, is stirring within them.

A Swedish study by Nils Uddenberg[3] and others confirmed findings that mild nausea during pregnancy is 'normal', but that severe vomiting indicates that the woman is probably undergoing severe stress, which may be for a variety of reasons. Uddenberg found that women who suffer mild nausea are the ones who are best adjusted to the female role and to their pregnancies. They were more likely to have planned their pregnancies than either the women with no nausea or the women with severe vomiting. The more sick the mothers the more this indicated a feeling that sex was disgusting. In common with some other studies, Uddenberg found that severe vomiting is linked to a masculine body build.[4] We do not know whether this is because 'masculine' women are constitutionally more likely to have psychological problems during pregnancy, or whether they have more psychological difficulty in accepting the feminine/female role. The second explanation seems much more likely.

Uddenberg also found that the group of women without any nausea at all showed signs that they were repressing the whole idea of pregnancy.

Adjusting to ambivalence

Good adjustment means adjusting to and accepting ambivalence. This idea is supported by a finding by Wolkind and Zajicek that six times as many of the women who did not vomit suffered definite psychiatric symptoms during the pregnancy. Of course such women were very much in the minority: a woman who does not suffer nausea need not assume that there must be something wrong with her.

If vomiting goes on for longer than the first three months, however, there may be something wrong with the environment, either physical or social.[5] Wolkind and Zajicek found that women whose vomiting lasted into the second or last three months were receiving less support than others from their own parents. They had poorer relationships with their own parents and saw them less frequently. (The study was done in an area of London where traditional family ties are still normally quite strong.) Although the husbands of those with a long-term problem had not expressed notably more hostile attitudes towards their wives' pregnancies, they were much less supportive of their wives in helping them to prepare, or preparing themselves for the coming of the baby.

Pre-eclampsia and toxaemia

The other common complication in pregnancy which appears to involve psychological stress is pre-eclampsia. This occurs in about 6 six per cent of all pregnancies in Europe and the USA, and, like vomiting, it is rare elsewhere, and quite unknown in some communities. The condition is characterised by raised blood pressure, oedema (a swelling of body and limbs caused by the collecting of water in the tissues), and protein in the urine.

In very rare cases, pre-eclampsia leads on to eclampsia, in which the three conditions are experienced to a much more serious degree, and the woman may suffer from convulsions. The condition is also known as toxaemia, dating from the time when the condition was mistakenly thought to be caused by some kind of blood poisoning.

The condition is probably caused by the interaction of physical and psychological factors. The bodily malfunction may be more likely in some women than in others because of their physical constitution. But in some cases at least it is triggered by a psychological event, or by her attitude to her pregnancy. (An analogy may be drawn with tuberculosis, which some persons are more likely to catch than others because of an inherited vulnerability, but which is precipitated by a bacterium.) It can occasionally be brought on in a normal pregnancy by sudden very severe stress. Pre-eclampsia usually goes with very high levels of anxiety during pregnancy, perhaps with other psychological disturbance, especially depression.

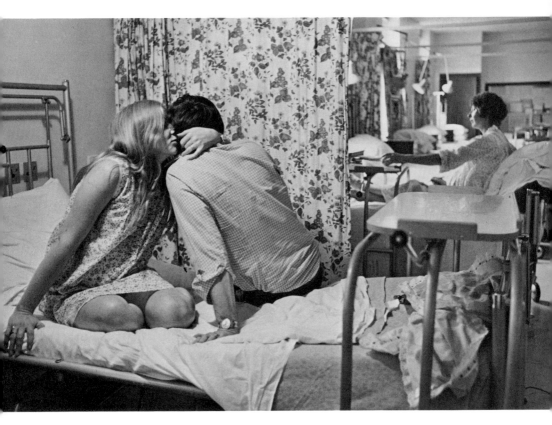

Like vomiting, pre-eclampsia can be associated with ambivalence and doubts about the pregnancy.[6] A. L. Coppen comments: 'the very fact of being pregnant [is] a considerable emotional disturbance in itself for many of these women'.[7] However there seems to be a difference in the origin of the psychological distress. Vomiting betokens problems to do with the coming child, whether they be in the mother-to-be's physical or social environment or in her readiness to care for the child. Pre-eclampsia seems to be associated more with the bodily challenge of being pregnant, with the woman's attitude to herself and her readiness to bear the body within her. However, further research is needed to clarify this.

Menstrual difficulties

Women who suffer from pre-eclampsia are more likely to have had difficulties over menstruation than other women. Many of the women that Coppen studied had never been told by their mothers—or anyone else—about menstruation, and were quite unprepared for it when it happened. Even those that had been told were more likely to have been shocked by it, and to go for longer than normal before their second menstruation. Coppen found that women with normal pregnancies were more likely to remember their first periods with reactions like 'I felt a woman at last', 'I felt grown up' or 'It seemed quite natural.' Women with pre-eclampsia, however, were more likely to say things like 'It was horrible', 'I felt as though I had cut myself', or 'I didn't tell my mother because I thought she would punish me.'

'The commonest attitude [of pre-eclampsic women] towards the menarche [starting menstruation],' says Coppen, 'and indeed to their menstrual periods later on, was one of resentment.' Not surprisingly, among these women there is much more premenstrual tension than normal, and also more sexual dysfunction. Pre-eclampsia seems to be more common among women who fail to achieve orgasm, or suffer from vaginal cramps and pain during intercourse, or simply find no pleasure in sex.

Most women are able to cope quite well with the great psychological tasks imposed on them by our cultural inheritance: the ignorance, confusion and suppression of women's physical and psychological nature. Those with psychosomatic complications in pregnancy are the minority who are less able to meet the extreme demands of self-sufficiency which are imposed upon them, and which in fact no one should be called upon to meet. Their problems are different not in kind but only in extent from those that face the rest of us.

9 Preparing for birth: pain and childbirth classes

We have concentrated so far on the psychology of pregnancy, its cultural setting and the process of adaptation that a woman must go through. There is, however, a quite separate source of stress, and that is the birth that ends the pregnancy.

One hundred years ago, childbirth was a fairly dangerous business for both parties. At its peak in the nineteenth century in England and Wales, six maternal deaths were recorded for each 1,000 births. The risk in hospitals from infection was even greater. One hospital recorded 33 deaths from infection per 1,000 births. In 1935 the maternal death rate started to fall and it has continued to decline dramatically. By 1971, the rate in England and Wales had dropped to 0.17 per 1,000. Most of these deaths either followed on abortions or were caused by medical conditions such as heart disease which had nothing to do with the pregnancy.[1]

How much unstated awareness of these historical risks remains in women's culture it is difficult to estimate. At least some women who were themselves born in 1935 are still bearing children. Folkways such as would embody such attitudes take years, possibly centuries to die out.

Mortality risk aside, however, childbirth is still a big, mysterious event. Apart from freak achievements during emergencies, it is probably the hardest work performed by humans. It is not called labour for nothing. And yet, until recently, the exact nature of the work to be done, and how it was achieved, was concealed. Indeed, even the word 'labour' was not used in polite society. A woman was 'confined', or 'brought to bed'— terms lacking any specific meaning, one carrying overtones of imprisonment, the other of illness.

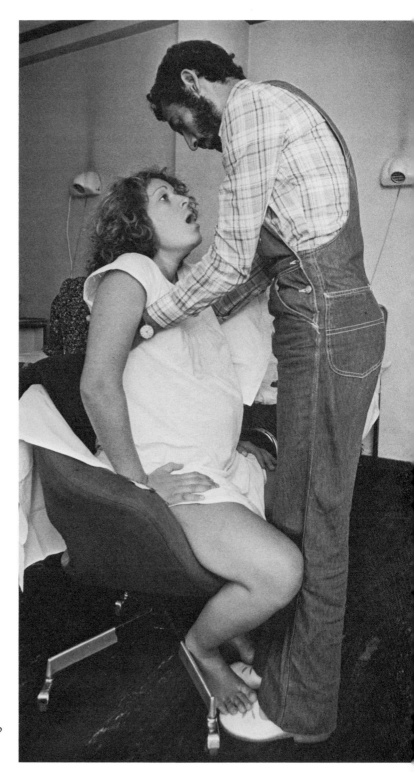

Not for nothing is the birth process called 'labour'—but Catherine Girardot has her husband Pierre to help with 'the hardest work performed by humans'.

89

The problem of pain

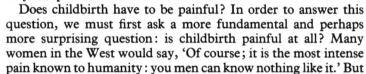

There is also the question of pain. There is an unspoken rule among women that one does not tell a first-timer what to expect, so as not to terrify her in advance. On the other hand, there is an opposite feeling that it is not fair to let a woman arrive at her first delivery in complete ignorance. The result, as one woman put it, is 'you try to let them know without actually telling them'. Medical staff may collude in this, and some standard hospital or clinic antenatal classes gloss over the subject. By this we do not mean that they ignore it, but that they may deal with it simply in terms of the methods of technological prevention by gas, or injection. At the same time old-fashioned nurses talk about 'the pains', enquiring in labour 'how often are the pains coming?'

The result is a confused state of half-knowledge. Many women who arrive in labour without benefit of good childbirth classes are utterly unprepared for what happens to them. A feeling of unreality often results. 'This can't be happening to me' may be the prevailing feeling and thought—hardly good auguries for the easy acceptance of motherhood afterwards.

Does childbirth have to be painful? In order to answer this question, we must first ask a more fundamental and perhaps more surprising question: is childbirth painful at all? Many women in the West would say, 'Of course; it is the most intense pain known to humanity: you men can know nothing like it.' But

At the Clinique des Lilas, the husband is a vital member of the delivery team: the advent of a new member is a shared family experience rather than a surgical procedure on an unconscious patient.

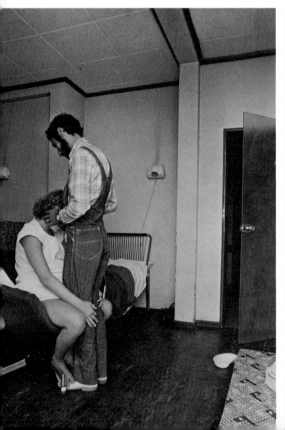
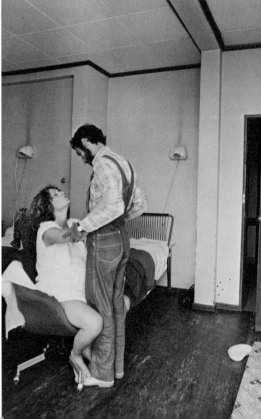

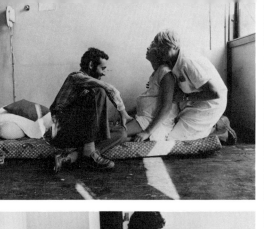
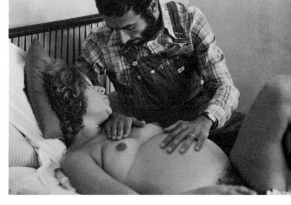
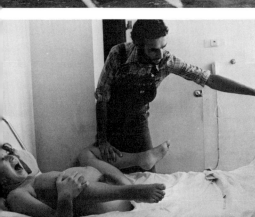
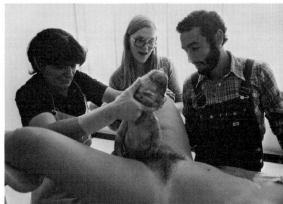
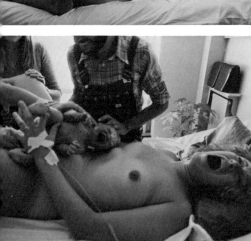
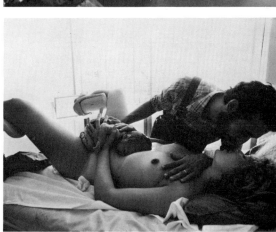
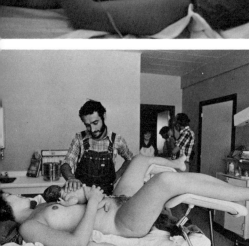
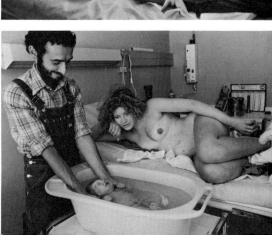

the British pioneer doctor Grantly Dick Read[2] was alerted to the possibility of painless childbirth when he encountered a woman in labour in London who felt no pain at all. It was she who told him that this was how childbirth should be.

In many societies women apparently do not feel pain as such. In some societies, where *couvade* is practised, the father is the one who retires to a darkened hut and groans in pain, taking several days to recover, while his wife goes back to work soon after the birth.[3]

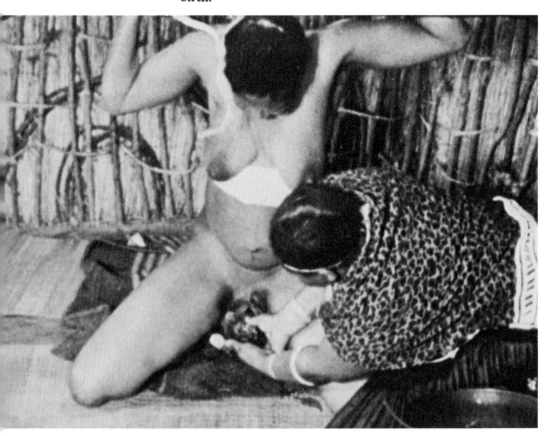

The sensations of birth are probably the same for all women: whether they are experienced as pain may depend largely on cultural expectations.

What is pain?

There can be no doubt that labour produces intense and utterly unfamiliar sensations in a woman. But are these pain? It is a well known psychological mechanism that when we are faced with something unknown or unfamiliar, we 're-create' it in our mind's eye in the likeness of something that we know and understand. In the West, we have only the very crudest language and concepts of bodily sensations to help us understand and express our internal experiences. A parallel may be found in the well known fact that the Eskimos have 16 words for different kinds of snow to our one. If we turn our minds to pain, we can begin to distinguish different kinds of pain.

Robert Melzack and W. S. Togerson found that feelings of pain vary in many ways. Light pain may flicker or quiver. Moderate pain may pulse and throb. Severe pain may beat or pound. Some pains jump, others flash or shoot. Some prick, others stab, both are different from cutting. Pinching, pressing, cramping and crushing are different yet again, and so are burning, scalding or searing pains. The feelings that these different kinds of pain produce also vary. The pains can produce feelings of numbness, of tension, of tiredness, sickness or suffocation and emotions of fear and punishment. But we have only one word to cover them all—pain. We even use the word pain to cover emotions like grief or disappointment.

And this is the word traditionally used in English to refer to the sensations of labour—whatever they are. By contrast, for example, Hebrew has one word for pain, *ka'ev* and a quite different word for the sensations of labour, *tsirim*, for which the easiest, though not exact, English translation would be contractions. So while some women regard the modern trend to use the word 'contractions' instead of 'labour pains' as a confidence trick, it makes perfectly good sense in Hebrew to enquire, 'are your *tsirim* giving you *ka'ev*?' because the two sensations are kept quite distinct.

The 'pain' we do not notice

It seems probable that all the time our bodies are registering something—perhaps we could call it subliminal pain—which in the normal course of events we do not feel or notice. But if we did not have this function, we would be in a bad way.

A case has been described of a girl who felt no pain at all. Not only did she suffer repeatedly from various kinds of wounds of which she had no sensation; but her bones and joints deteriorated: her failure to register discomfort subliminally caused her to use her frame and limbs far more severely than is normal. Most of us protect ourselves by moderating our movements and shifting position to lessen and distribute the loads on our bodies. But in the normal course of events, we would not describe what we feel as pain.

The level at which these unconscious warning signals become consciously interpreted—as pain or some other sensation—vary widely from culture to culture and from individual to individual. In one experiment, levels of heat stimulation that Northern Europeans experienced as 'warm' produced pain in persons of Mediterranean origin. In another, women of Italian origin refused to tolerate levels of electric shock that were accepted easily by Anglo-Saxon and Jewish women. It has also been found that Jewish women respond better to suggestion than Protestant women. When they were told that their religious group had a poor tolerance of pain, their levels of tolerance rose, while the Protestant women's tolerance was unaffected.

At a more dramatic level, well documented reports from many societies all over the world describe men in religious ecstasies or 'rites of passage' inflicting serious wounds on themselves without apparent feelings of pain. They recover with striking rapidity and their wounds heal quickly, leaving little or no scarring. Many men who are wounded in war at the time experience little or no pain from quite severe wounds.[4] Surgery patients who are giving or receiving a kidney in a transplant operation have been found to experience pain to different degrees and in different patterns from those patients having 'general' surgery, such as a hysterectomy.

Letting pain through

To explain these phenomena, Robert Melzack and Patrick Wall produced their 'gate' control theory of pain.[5] They suggest that there is a nervous mechanism which opens or closes a 'gate', controlling how much input from pain receptors reaches the brain. If the 'gate' opens wide, or stays partly open for some time, then enough input reaches the brain to produce the feelings of pain. The gate can be opened and closed by stimulation of appropriate nerves from other parts of the body. (This is how acupuncture works.)

The operation of this gate is also affected by psychological processes. Anxiety can increase pain, and a person's attitudes to events can determine whether or not he feels pain.

But the amount of pain felt at the time of a particular experience is not the only important factor. Reactions to pain can vary immensely. For instance, 'Old' Americans and the British tend to keep their feelings to themselves. They withdraw when in pain and cry out or moan only in private. Jews and Italians are much more expressive and tend to seek support and sympathy. Jews and Italians also differ from each other: Italians usually direct their priorities to relief and escape from the pain; Jews tend to want to understand its meaning and implications. (These are the findings of a study of how people actually behave. If they seem like familiar stereotypes, that just shows that there is some truth in some stereotypes.)[6]

Not a method that would recommend itself to modern obstetricians; but no worse than some of the procedures in use until quite recently in more 'enlightened' societies.

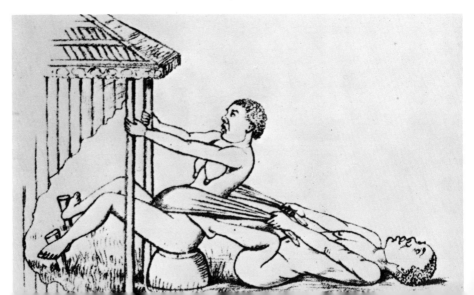

Sybil Eysenck found that women experience pain in labour differently according to their personalities.[7] Although extroverts normally experience pain less than introverts, it was the extroverts who complained more of pain and said that they had had a hard labour. The nurses, however, did not think there had been much difference between extroverts and introverts.

Pain, fear and ignorance

Grantly Dick Read first suggested the 'triad' of pain in childbirth, in which the anticipation and fear of pain produces anxiety which in turn produces pain. According to Read, if fear could be removed, then the pain would disappear as well. Research on the nature of pain broadly supports this suggestion. If pain is anticipated, then anxiety levels rise and the experience of pain increases. Sensations which do not produce pain in some people are experienced as pain by others who expect them to be painful.

However, it is not the anticipation of pain which itself leads to pain. If it were, then the most effective way of avoiding pain would be to deny that it exists. In fact, denial beforehand actually increases pain, perhaps by producing a shock reaction to it. The real culprits are fear and ignorance.

It has been clearly established that when a patient has some knowledge of a surgical operation and its aftermath, when he is told roughly how much pain and what kind of pain he can anticipate, then the experience of pain is reduced, and the stress he suffers is also lower.[8]

Childbirth pain has an added dimension: it is likely to be more severe in women who are negative or ambivalent about their pregnancy. Studies in Sweden have shown that the women who have the most pain in birth are on the whole those who have had the most psychological disturbance during pregnancy. This includes those with most marital problems, those who are reluctant to tell their own mothers about the coming baby, and women who are late in contacting their antenatal clinic.[9] Women in this category tended to show little interest in caring for the child after it was born, and to want either no more children or small families. These women had often used unreliable contraception and had passively 'let themselves get pregnant'.

Training for childbirth

Childbirth classes have been found to be a help, in that they teach women about pregnancy and motherhood. They are also given an opportunity to discuss with the teacher and with other mothers-to-be their doubts and attitudes, and to see their own position in relation to that of other women.

Preventing pain

A number of experiments have investigated the effect of the psychoprophylactic (meaning psychological preventative, and known as PPM) techniques used in childbirth or other kinds of pain.[10] The news is, they work. Marie Bobey and P. O. Davidson compared the effectiveness of 'cognitive rehearsal', that is, going over in the mind what is to come, with a general relaxation programme. Both were found to increase pain tolerance, although relaxation was generally more effective.[11]

In a very thorough experiment R. J. Stevens and F. Heide compared different techniques and combinations of techniques.[12] First they gave a group simple relaxation training. A second group received 'feedback relaxation', that is, the instructor came round and, by lifting an arm or leg, showed them how relaxed they were becoming, so that they could practise further if necessary. Some members of these two groups were then taught 'attention focus'. This is an important ingredient in psycho-prophylaxis, in which the woman concentrates her attention on some feature of her environment, such as a spot on the wall or a light switch, in order to direct it from the unwelcome sensations. Another group was taught attention focus on its own without relaxation, and a final control group was taught nothing. Each volunteer had to keep her hand in a bucket of ice-water for as long as she could stand, up to a maximum of four minutes, take it out and warm it up in water at blood heat, and then immerse it again, four times. So the experiment made at least an attempt to mimic the coming and dying away of labour contractions.

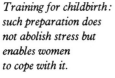

Training for childbirth: such preparation does not abolish stress but enables women to cope with it.

The volunteers who tolerated the pain best were those whose training was most like PPM—those who had had attention focus and relaxation with feedback. Among the other volunteers, the less training received the lower the pain tolerance. A striking finding was that for all those with training, the tolerance levels went up with each new immersion, and the more training the

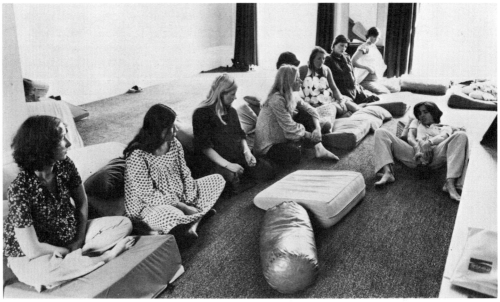

greater the rise. But the group who had had no training at all were able to tolerate less and less pain each time.

It has been suggested that the beneficial effects claimed for childbirth training are due not to the training itself, but to the personalities of the women who go to classes, or to their higher levels of motivation.[13] However, studies have shown that although motivation does affect the childbirth experiences of women and their relationship with their babies after the birth, it is not as important as the classes themselves.[14]

The influence of education

A woman's level of education seems to be a factor as well. Many studies in different countries have found that the lower the level of education a woman achieves the more pain she is likely to feel in childbirth. It would be easy to confuse educational level with social class here, as on the whole it is lower-class women who are less well educated. Class in itself does not seem to make a difference in birth pain. It is lack of education and the life stress caused by bad housing and poor social conditions that matter. Why this should be, we do not yet know. It could be that

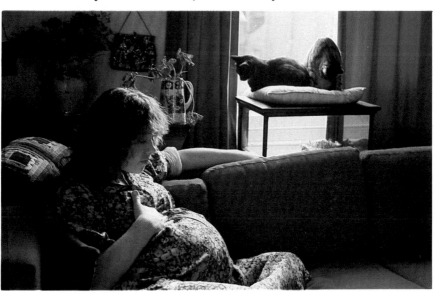

Waiting—perhaps wondering whether it will be painful: fear and ignorance will make it worse.

education brings with it a general ability to cope with stress. It could be that education confers self-esteem, which increases pain tolerance. It is also among the poorest educated women that one meets with the attitude: 'I don't want to know anything about it: just get the baby out and get it over with.' This attitude very commonly leads to long labour with much pain.

The effects of training

One of the most comprehensive studies of the effects of actively preparing for childbirth was undertaken by Susan Doering and Doris Entwisle,[15] who studied 269 American women who were all married and living with their husbands. Half had taken a full

97

course in psychoprophylaxis, and half had had other kinds of preparation in varying degrees, from no preparation at all to quite thorough preparation.

Level one contained those women who had had no training, and who said things like 'I didn't want to know *anything*.' At level two were those women who had read books and magazines about pregnancy and birth and who knew about the psychology involved, but who had not attended classes and did not know about coping techniques. At level three were those women who had level two knowledge, plus some knowledge of psychophysical techniques. This group included those who attended classes based on Grantly Dick Read's methods and philosophy. Level four was composed of the women who had had a full PPM training (Lamaze in this case).

It was found that the more training the mother had, the more aware and conscious she was likely to be at birth.

Among women with full psychoprophylactic training, a striking 84 per cent were fully conscious and only five per cent unconscious. Even a small degree of preparation—such as that achieved by women at level two—was enough to increase the proportion who were partly conscious or aware from 37 per cent to 69 per cent: although only 4 per cent of these women managed to remain conscious and aware throughout.

(It is only in the USA that such very high rates of general anaesthesia apply. Elsewhere it is used only for caesarian sections and very difficult forceps deliveries, in 5 to 10 per cent of women at most. How much medication a woman receives in childbirth is strongly influenced by the policy in the unit where she is giving birth. Some will allow her complete freedom of choice, but many will wish to apply their own standards.)

Training and attitude to birth
Does it really matter whether a woman is conscious or not? Doering and Entwisle confirm other findings; women who receive training benefit from it afterwards, as do their babies. They go further, however, and show that it is the level of consciousness and awareness during the birth which largely produces these good results. The more aware the mothers, the more positive their feelings about the experience of childbirth later. One of the justifications for anaesthetics during delivery is that the whole process is so ghastly and even frightening, that women are better off without any knowledge of it. This is shown to be wrong.

Simple learning theory psychology might suggest that the pain and anxiety that is expected during delivery might condition the mother adversely and turn her against it. The results, however, show that the opposite is true. Fifty-seven per cent of the women who were completely unconscious during the birth felt negatively about it afterwards, and only 3 per cent felt positively. Ninety-one per cent of those who were fully conscious felt positively, while only 3 per cent felt negatively.

The results for the baby

Perhaps even more important, mothers' attitudes to their babies were similarly affected. Fifty-nine per cent of those who had been completely unconscious had a negative reaction. Of the fully conscious women, only 8 per cent had a negative reaction, while 81 per cent had a positive reaction.

These attitudes had an effect on how the baby was cared for. Of the mothers who had positive attitudes from the start, 59 per cent breast-fed their babies for more than six months, compared with only 20 per cent of the mothers with negative attitudes. Of the negative mothers, 51 per cent did not even attempt to breast-feed, but only 9 per cent of the positive mothers bottle-fed entirely. Positive mothers were also much more likely to keep their babies with them in hospital instead of allowing them to be taken away to a nursery.

When a woman 'fails'

Some women arrive at labour with all that they have read or been taught about natural childbirth in their minds, and determined to go through with it without anaesthetic. Then during the labour they find the pain more than they think they can stand and accept an anaesthetic injection or a spinal block.

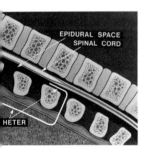

If pain becomes intolerable, it can be 'blocked' by anaesthetics administered spinally.

After the birth, many women who have changed their minds in this way feel remorseful and consider that they have failed. The tendency then is to comfort the woman, and to reassure her by denying her feeling of having lost control. It is doubtful whether this is wise. Much the better course is to allow the woman to accept that she has failed the target she set herself, but to examine whether it was a real target in the first place. If the pain in the end did reach intolerable levels, then the target moved, and her original intention was outdated. No woman can predict in advance how much pain she is going to feel. But it is more helpful for her to come to terms with this than to pretend she never really intended to do without anaesthetics.

On the other hand, perhaps she never really did intend to do without them. Many women arrive at labour with all sorts of feelings of what they ought to do or ought not to do, and not always with the training to go with those ideas. If a woman's intention to do without drugs was really only lip-service to ideals which she did not genuinely share herself, then it is going to be more useful to her to be allowed the chance to re-examine her ideals than merely to be soothed down.

A third possibility is that the woman is playing the game, 'See What You Made Me Do.' Many of us do this. When we cannot make up our minds, we act in a way that encourages others to take the decision for us. Once someone has done this, we can react in two ways. We can go with the decision and be grateful towards those that helped us in our dilemma, or we can claim that we 'really' wanted to take the other course and that the choice was forced on us.

10   Mother and baby

It is done. With the aid of a doctor or a midwife, and one hopes of your husband, you have delivered a new child into the world. Not a nugget of gold, nor an ingot of cast iron, but an alive and alert human being.

The aware baby

Alert? Much of what is done to babies in the first few days or weeks of their lives is done on the assumption that they are largely unaware of what is going on around them. One of the most common questions that new mothers ask is, 'Can my baby see?'

Until very recently the answer she would have had from nearly everybody was either 'No' or 'Not very much'. Even now, many women believe that newborn babies are blind and deaf, and many midwives and some doctors will still tell them so. Other myths that survive among both women and medical staff is that babies cannot remember anything that happens to them, and that they cannot feel pain. The first three of these are certainly wrong, and the last *almost* certainly so.

Within two or three minutes of birth most babies who are born normally and without heavy anaesthetics are looking round them. When their eyes fall upon a bright stimulus they will stare at it. If their eyes fall on a nearby human face they will fix upon it and gaze steadily. A few weeks later babies explore the features of a face more positively. Experiments show that their recognition of complex artificial stimuli improves early and steadily. In the past, psychologists have also assumed that the abilities of new babies are very limited. Without any evidence quite blunt assertions have been made that new babies cannot do this, that and the other.

These assertions have been proved wrong. The developmental psychologist Harry McGurk has pointed out how difficult it is to obtain reliable information from laboratory experiments on babies.[1] Because a baby does not do what the experimenter wants, that does not mean that he *cannot* do it. It may be that the conditions are not right, or that he is just not interested.

The baby after birth
Recent research by Deborah Rosenblatt, Martin Packer and Margaret Redshaw found that after birth a typical baby gives a

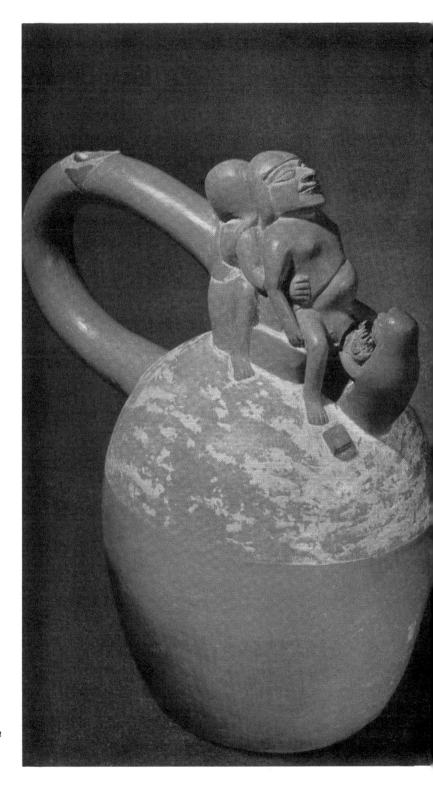

*The process of birth
has always been much
the same—but for each
new mother it
is still unique.*

short 'birth cry' and then settles into a quiet, semi-alert state, interspersed with brief periods of full alertness.[2] He will 'fuss' a good deal, but cry only a little. He is not likely to sleep unless, perhaps, he is having a little trouble in breathing. He is probably very changeable, switching from fussiness to crying, to being semi-alert, then to fully alert and back again very often and quickly. A good deal of the baby's crying in this study was in response to handling by hospital staff in 'aversive' tests and routines that the baby finds unpleasant.

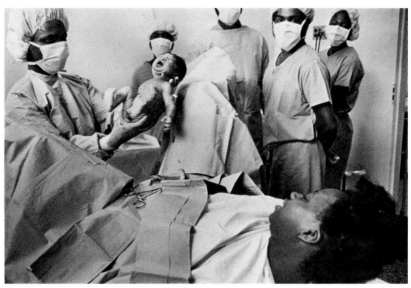

The cry of life—and already the baby is a fully functional human being.

On their first day of life the babies spent an average of seven hours awake. After the first day this dropped sharply and only reached seven hours again after a week.

At birth just under 90 per cent of the babies could follow the face of someone who was talking to them at the same time as the face moved back and forth. They found that easier than tracking a shiny object like a necklace. Nevertheless, more than four-fifths could manage the latter task also.

Babies have usually been said to be deaf at birth because it is assumed (apparently without any evidence) that the eustachian tubes that connect the middle ear to the throat are blocked. This means that the ear remains full of amniotic fluid from the womb. One teacher in the London Hospital used to say that if one were lucky one could sometimes see an expression of amazement pass over the face of a baby during the first week as his eustachian tubes cleared and he heard for the first time.

In fact, although water in the tubes would certainly muffle hearing, producing an effect like heavy catarrh, it would not make the baby completely deaf. So we need not be surprised at Rosenblatt's finding that at birth nine-tenths of the babies she studied would alert or turn their eyes when a rattle was shaken to one side of them; and that more than a third turned their heads towards the sound. A day after birth, nearly two-thirds turned towards the sound.

How the baby knows his mother

Carefully performed experiments done in conditions coming close to real life or studies of babies in different everyday care have shown the following facts, unimaginable a few years ago. By two to three weeks most babies, if they have been breast-fed, can distinguish their mothers from any other person by smell.[3] They can recognise their mother's voice—if they have had free access to her.[4] Most importantly, perhaps, they can recognise their

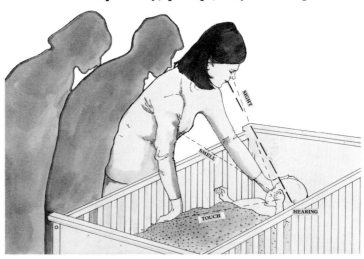

Babies very quickly come to distinguish their mothers from other people.

mother's face, in normal circumstances, from any other, and from a mask.[5] If a baby is cared for in hospital by a nurse on a regular basis so that he is able to grow accustomed to her style, he notices when a new caretaker takes over, and may be distressed by the change.[6]

All these facts mean that not only is a two-to-three-week-old baby very much more aware of his environment than was formerly thought, but that he must be aware and learning from very early in life. There is no reason, indeed, to suppose that he does not begin to learn the moment he is born, since he can certainly learn before he is born, as experiments showed many years ago. Deborah Rosenblatt believes that three-day-old babies have already started adjusting to the behaviour of their caretakers and their physical environment.

If a baby does not show the abilities we have described until he is two or three weeks old his mother need not conclude that there is something wrong with him. Some babies develop more slowly than others. However, it is important to note that medical intervention in birth can have an adverse effect on the baby.[7]

Pain-killers and anaesthetics taken by the mother during birth all pass through the placenta to the baby in greater or lesser amounts. This can result in a baby who is irritable, and less good than others at becoming alert and responding to particular stimuli. Perhaps because of this, many babies do not establish good feeding patterns for some time. The use of forceps may have a similar effect, and has also been linked with jaundice. (Forceps are used five times as frequently in induced as in 'natural' births. In about 10 per cent of births, however, these risks may be outweighed by advantages in induction.) This is another great advantage of psychoprophylactic classes, for they lead to lower amounts of medication, or none at all, and can help a mother to avoid the need to accelerate a slow labour with medication. Moreover, a woman who is offered an induction that she does not want may find it easier to refuse if she is well prepared.

The 'bond' between mother and baby

Is there a natural or instinctive bond between the new baby and his mother? Much has been made of this idea in recent years.

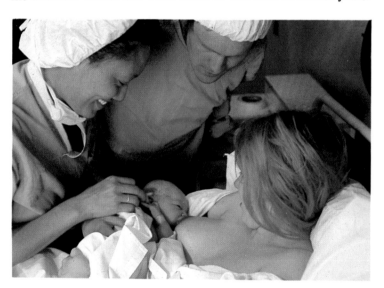

'Breast fed is best fed.'

Unfortunately, however, the discussion has been characterised by more heat than light. Most people are fervently devoted to one side or the other. Sceptics refuse to consider the possibility of any such relationship; while believers teach that any disturbance of the links between mother and child can damage the child psychologically for life.

A third group, of which the psychiatrist Michael Rutter is one, believe that the bond does not develop until the baby is six months old.[8] This is presumably because that is the age at which the baby becomes aware that objects continue to exist even when he cannot see them. But that is something different—it is an awareness of the concept of things. In fact we know now that as early as two weeks after birth a baby is aware when his routine is

104

changed and he 'knows' his mother—if he is given the chance to get to know her.

Unfortunately, we simply do not have the information that would enable us to say whether this 'knowledge' influences the rest of the baby's life. One or two studies suggest that changes such as abrupt weaning at the age of three months, which amounts to a complete change in the baby's experience of his mother, can lead to behavioural and emotional problems later in life.[9] Recently developed regression techniques in psychotherapy support this idea. But we have nothing to match the studies which show the damage that can be caused by some separations at two years; or the complete lack of emotional caretaking that used to be found in some institutions.

There is, however, more evidence to show a 'bonding' effect in the other direction, of the mother to the child. Animal experiments and natural observation show that in many species, if the young are removed from their mother for a short period soon after birth, she rejects them completely when they are

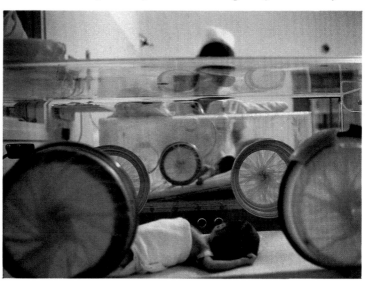

'... ripp'd untimely from my mother's womb ...' and popped, for salvation, into this mechanical womb, the incubator.

returned. Yet it is still standard practice in many hospitals to remove babies soon after birth. Since we are human, we are usually able to overcome the rejection effects that such régimes can produce. But not always.

When mothers have complete freedom

In a classic study, Marshall Klaus and John Kennel gave a group of mothers a period of unlimited contact with their babies immediately after birth.[10] They left mother and child together on the bed. The baby was naked, and a special heat panel above the bed kept him warm. The mothers laid their babies on the bed beside them so that they could look into each other's eyes. Then, talking to him softly began to explore the baby gently with her hands. Using first the tips of her fingers, then the whole length

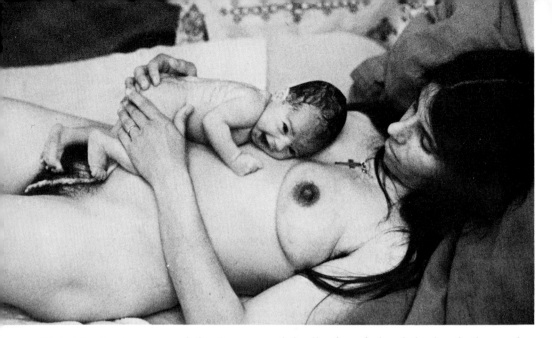

*Births following the
Leboyer methods, in
which the mother and
baby are left in gentle
intimacy, can produce
lasting benefits in the
child's development.*

of the fingers, and finally the whole of the hand, the mother moved from a most tentative touching to a firm but gentle massage of the baby's whole body. When these babies were older, their mothers were still taking more time and trouble over caring for them. They were doing this more lovingly than mothers whose babies had been removed from them in standard American hospital fashion. In some cases the mother had also given the breast to the baby, and the effect on these mothers was even more pronounced. These mothers were not taught what to do: they were left entirely to do what they wanted. The common pattern suggests strongly that it is 'instinctive', or guided by natural inborn tendencies.

A repeat of this study in a hospital in England by Andrew Whiten produced a similarly more loving attitude in those mothers given completely free access to their babies after the birth.[11] After six months, however, the difference between these mothers and a comparison group given standard treatment had disappeared. We do not know whether this was because the standardly treated mothers had caught up, or because the specially treated mothers had slipped back under the pressure of normal life. The difference between Whiten's mothers and those studied by Klaus and Kennel is that the English women were middle class, while the South American women were socially very disadvantaged.

In England, too, there is a more permissive attitude towards mothers and babies, although access is not always unrestricted. The effects found by Klaus and Kennel, then, are partly the effect of contrast with the extreme practice in American hospitals. More importantly, middle class mothers who are able to take their babies home to a good environment and to middle class culture are able to compensate for their early inadequate experience of their babies. The question is, is compensation good enough? And are we right to continue on the basis that mothers can compensate, since not all can?

A wealth of evidence shows that the better a mother's attitude to her child at birth, the better the quality of her care-giving throughout the rest of his childhood. Children who are removed from their mothers are at risk of being battered if other factors (such as class and social stress) also lead in the same direction. They are also more likely, with the same contribution from class and stress, to become delinquent.

The first few hours after the birth form a critical period for mother and probably child. We should therefore do our utmost to take advantage of that fact, and not interfere with the establishment of the basic relationship.

We must add a big BUT here, however. Human powers of adaptation and recovery are impressive, as we have said. A mother who has not been able to have access to her child after the birth, either because of the practice of the hospital she is in or because the baby has needed intensive care, should not feel doomed. She can make it up to herself and her baby if her circumstances favour this.

Feeding the baby

Many books on child care hedge their bets on the subject of breast- or bottle-feeding. The advice given is often highly equivocal: 'Breast is best but the bottle is just as good' is usually the message. This probably reflects two things. First, most such books are written by doctors who are trying to find a way of expressing in a single text all the variety of advice that they are called upon to give to mothers from many different backgrounds and with many different problems (or no problems).

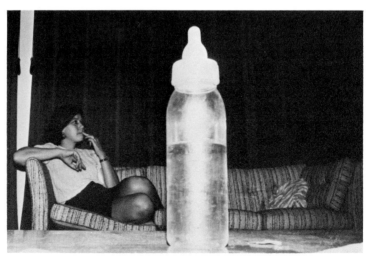

The 'breast v bottle' argument may loom large in the young mother's life.

107

Secondly, it is important that a woman should not be made to breast-feed when she does not want to, since most of its psychological advantages would thus be negated. So she should not be made to feel guilty for deciding to bottle feed. Also in the background is the awareness that many women who choose not to breast-feed later wish that they had done so. It is felt, too, that these women should not be made to feel guilty.

Perhaps the best approach, therefore, is to give information rather than advice to mothers. Every woman must make up her own mind and choose what she thinks will be best for herself and her child. When we say, then, that we firmly believe that, all other things being equal, breast is best, we must immediately add that we are well aware that other things rarely are equal. It is the importance of those 'other things' to her and her child that a mother must assess for herself to guide her choice between breast and bottle.

Breast is best

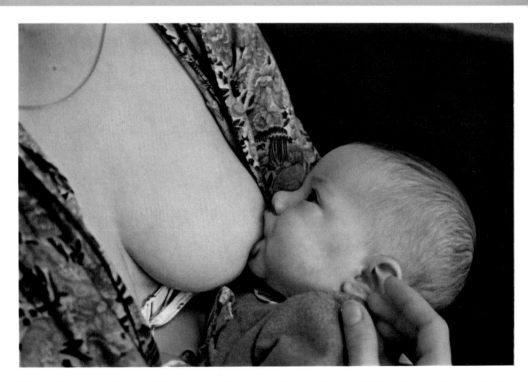

'Food, glorious food!'

Why do we think that breast is best? We will deal first with the biomedical reasons.[12] The colostrum that the breasts give out in the first two or three days after the birth is a clearish liquid of variable, though usually yellowish, colour. It is rich in protein and antibodies that help to protect the baby against infection.

Human milk itself has been 'designed' by human evolution to suit the baby's stomach. Its make-up is very different from that of dried milk formulae. In particular, it has a different balance of types of protein, making it much more easily digestible. What is more, the make-up of the milk changes during the course of the feed, which a bottle cannot do.

Then there are psychological advantages. First, there is the simple increase in body contact between mother and child. Research with monkeys (because we could not treat human babies in the brutal way needed to test such theories) shows that touch and contact is more important to a baby than feeding in forming a relationship with the mother. It provides the self-confidence needed later to deal with threat and anxiety.

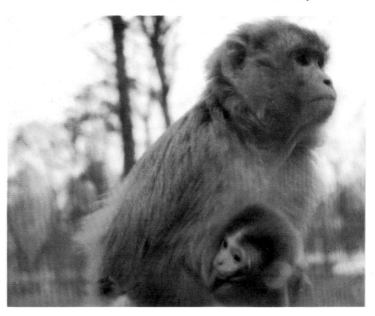

That is why we are all called 'mammals'.

Second, there is the increased eye-contact. A baby's eyes have a resting focus of the same length as an adult's, about 200mm (8 ins). This corresponds roughly with the average distance between a baby's eyes and his mother's face when she is breast-feeding him. Mothers who breast-feed are likely to spend more time bent over their child in direct eye-contact. They also tend to smile more at their babies.

Third, there is soothing and caressing. Mothers who breast-feed tend to spend more time caressing and stroking their babies. This is not just because they are not holding a bottle in one hand : most tend to use their free hand to manipulate the breast to help the flow of milk and stimulate the baby's mouth area. The hand with which they hold the baby caresses it as well.

Fourth, there is increased vocal communication. Breast-feeding mothers spend more time talking to their babies. The talk tends to be more affectionate, too.

Letting the baby take charge

What all this amounts to is more and better communication between mother and child. Psychologists now lay emphasis on 'contingent responding', in which one person's actions produce results in the form of reactions or adaptation by others. Depression is known to go with a loss of 'contingent responding', and is also influenced by experiences in early childhood. So it is obviously desirable to give a child experience of contingent responding early in life. Breast-feeding does this. Perhaps because of the greater scope for communication between mother and child and because of its greater sensitivity, mothers and breast-fed babies settle more quickly into a stable feeding routine in which each adjusts to the other. What is more, the baby has more control over the feeding process, and is much more likely than his bottle-fed contemporary to decide when he has had enough. Mothers who bottle-feed are more likely than breast-feeders to remove the teat and end the feed, or to insist that the baby carries on until the 'right' amount has been taken.

One study found that women whose mothers had breast-fed them when they were babies were better adjusted behaviourally as adults if their mother had been warm to them, while those whose mothers had been cold adjusted less well. Women who had been bottle-fed were not so much influenced by their mothers' attitudes.

Bottle feeding

The arguments in favour of bottle-feeding focus on a woman's way of life, on her feelings about breast-feeding and on her career choice. Although breast-feeding is more convenient than bottle-feeding, in that the milk is always ready and needs no special equipment, it is true that a mother who wants to breast-feed successfully will have to lead a quieter life than she could allow herself if she were bottle-feeding. If she returns to paid work—or leads a generally unrelaxed life—she may find that her milk dries up. Of course, there are exceptions. Many women have worked and breast-fed—sometimes in the same place— quite successfully.

A woman who is unhappy with her baby can inhibit the baby's feeding, making him more distressed and slowing down his development. This is a good reason why women who feel strongly averse to breast-feeding should probably either bottle-feed, or explore the reasons for their feelings.[13] That leads us to an aspect of the feeding question that is not normally considered in guides on baby management. Attitudes to breast-feeding are not entirely separate from attitudes to pregnancy and birth. Some women who bottle-feed do so because they do not like the strong bodily feelings involved in breast-feeding. And we have already seen that if a woman is not happy with her body she is more likely to have an unhappy time in pregnancy and complications in birth.

Some studies have actually found that a woman's intention early in pregnancy to breast-feed indicates that she is more likely to have a relatively problem-free pregnancy and birth. This seems to tie up with the finding that a mother who considers her unborn baby as a person early in pregnancy is more likely to form a good relationship with him after the birth.

Hindrances to breast feeding

Only about 1 per cent of women are physically incapable of breast-feeding. However, the psychological environment in the first days after the birth strongly influences the success with which breast-feeding is established. Niles Newton believes that humans evolved to make love, give birth and feed babies unobtrusively in quiet surroundings because our forebears would otherwise have been most at risk from predators at those times. This would explain why anxiety can inhibit all three processes.

The presence of other people seems to be a potent cause of anxiety in mothers breast-feeding for the first time. Even when others are trying to help the mother, their interference can have the opposite effect. Dr Peter de Chateau found in Sweden that the act of weighing a baby each day, however well the baby is doing, tends to put a mother off breast-feeding (and supplementary feeds help to put the baby off). He also found that support from the father helps a woman breast-feed.[14]

Another common cause of mothers' giving up breast-feeding is their anxiety about their own capacity to nourish the baby. These women assume that each time their baby cries it is a cry of hunger, resulting from their own inadequacy as 'feeders'. This anxiety is almost always based on a woman's fantasy that she is inadequate for the role of mother. It has virtually nothing to do with the actual capacity of her breasts to produce milk. It is commonly associated with postnatal depression, which we will discuss in the next chapter.

However, it seems that once a mother is breast-feeding, she may be more resistant to stress and keep a more stable mood than a mother who is bottle-feeding or a woman not involved in child care at all.

The first rule of survival: keep hold of your food supply!

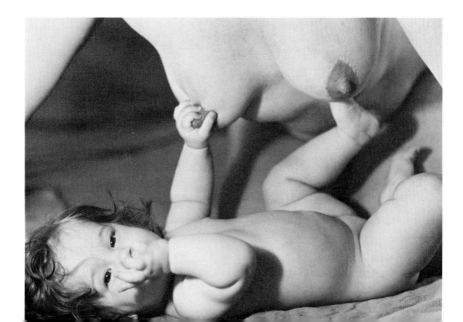

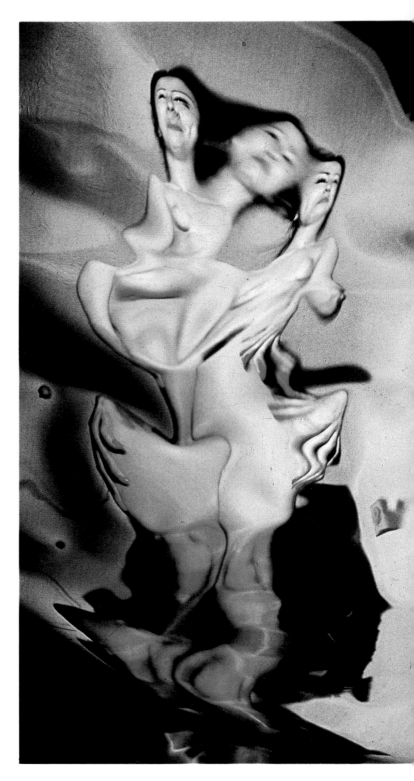

'... such a mixed-up
feeling after
I had the baby ...'

112

11 Depression and the blues

Many women who are fortunate enough to clear all the hurdles that traditional attitudes and hospital routines put in their way (and those who are lucky enough to be able to have their babies at home) find the period immediately after the birth a time of elation and ecstasy. Their joy and contentment is a pleasure and a wonder for others to see. Most people however have the impression that 'the blues'—post-natal depression—is more characteristic of women's mood after giving birth.

The blues

A period of tears and sorrow is quite normal. As many as four-fifths of mothers experience a brief period of tearfulness at some time during the first few days after the birth. Sometimes the mood creeps on slowly, and the mother may slide gently into a mood of doubt and sorrow, climbing as slowly and imperceptibly out of it after a few hours. More often, however, the onset is sudden. Many women are quite unprepared for it when it happens to them. A woman may be astonished to find herself bursting into tears without any apparent provocation at the moment when she 'should' be happy, such as when her husband arrives for a visit. Then, after perhaps as little a time as an hour, the mood is gone and all is sunshine again.

A much smaller proportion find themselves with a depression that may last a few weeks or months, or occasionally a year or two. Many of this second group do not realise what has happened to them. They feel changed, but are not able to put their finger on quite how. Their friends and husbands may notice a change, but they, too, may not know how to describe it. In a severe depression the total paralysis of will and feelings of despair are unmistakable. However, very few women indeed reach this level. More typically there is an indefinable lessening of drive, a slowing of pace, a feeling of slight helplessness and hopelessness. The sense of humour may diminish or disappear and interest and pleasure in sex may be low or nil.[1]

In the first few days some women find themselves confused and disoriented, feeling not quite sure who or where they are or wnat age. In a few women, this confusion is so intense that it can look like the thought-disorder and illusion that go with some kinds of schizophrenia. Except in a very tiny number of cases, these feelings pass after two or three weeks at the most, leaving only the depression.[2]

It is sad that many women do not recognise the change in them for what it is, for post-natal depression, or post partum syndrome, is usually quite easily dispersed with psychotherapy. If it is treated properly, it need hardly ever last very long—and it can often be avoided with proper preparation.

'Post partum syndrome'

Many theories have been put forward over the years to account for postnatal depression on physical grounds. Changes in hormones and body fluid levels have commonly been pointed to, and the condition has been treated as though it were an abnormality. One theory was that these changes affected the brain, producing delirium. Most recently, the sudden massive drop in the level of progesterone after the birth has been suggested as a possible cause. This may indeed be one of the contributory factors to the blues, which come so soon after the birth and last such a comparatively short time. But the connection has not been proved. The blues may equally be a normal reaction to a very intense psychological experience—a return to earth after a peak experience. Intellectual functions, such as short-term memory, are not affected.

There is probably a psychological reaction to hormonal and other physiological changes, similar to that described earlier in this book in the discussion of mood changes in pregnancy. Some confusion may also arise out of the very abrupt changes in the new mother's anatomy. Within a few hours, she loses most of her bulge, a good deal of weight, and her internal organs return to something like their original positions. She has not, however, fully returned to her state before pregnancy. Her womb and heart are larger, her general muscle tone lower, and she may retain a certain amount of fluid and body fat. When the milk first enters her breasts on about the third day after birth, they feel very strange—solid, hard, and sometimes sore. So having adapted for nine months to a new shape, that image is suddenly gone—but she is not her old self either.

Physical changes are not necessary, however, to produce post partum symptoms, which also occur in a few women who have adopted babies. These women show exactly the same mental confusion, anxiety and depression as biological mothers. Moreover, as we have already noted, some fathers also show signs of confusion and depression on the birth of their first child.

Several psychologists who have followed the whole process of pregnancy, birth and the months that follow stress the fact that birth is not a clean and sharp end to pregnancy. It is not, after all, a simple door through which one enters a new room immediately. During pregnancy and birth, an enormous mental shakedown takes place. Old ways of thought are loosened, broken up and discarded, with the greatest 'mind tremors' occurring in the hours after birth.

Although mental rehearsal during pregnancy gets her off to a flying start, a woman's new identity as a mother does not really begin to form until the baby is born and she can establish a real, as distinct from imaginary, relationship with him. Thus, in the days after the birth, a new mother is perhaps least in charge of herself. However, she is normally very active and ready to care for the child if allowed to do so. Sadly, there may be obstacles in her way, both in her psychological history and in her current surroundings.

'Learned helplessness'

A fruitful breakthrough in psychology in recent years has been the identification of depression with 'learned helplessness'.[3] The classic experiment is one in which animals are placed in a harness and then given electric shocks from which there is no escape. After a few such sessions, the animals are placed in a cage divided in two by a low barrier and with a grid in the floor through which they can be shocked on the feet. Normally, animals in this situation learn quickly to jump over the barrier to escape from the shock to the other side. Animals that have experienced inescapable shock, however, very rarely make their escape. Even when they do so, they seem incapable of learning from it. In the end, most of them lie down and accept the shock, to the point of actively resisting attempts to lead them away from the situation. The animals have learned to be helpless.

It now seems clear that humans can show the same changes in their behaviour and in their beliefs about what is possible when they suffer traumatic experiences from which they cannot escape. When these experiences happen, a temporary lowering of mood and behaviour may result which disappears in time. But several such traumas can produce a more permanent change, in which the person whose ability to act and to learn is seriously disrupted.

Recent research in London by a team of sociologists led by George Brown has shown that depression in women in a large city is linked with four 'vulnerability factors'.[4] The depression itself is usually brought on by a 'life event', a loss or a change involving stress, such as bereavement, separation or divorce or moving home, or long-term stress from poor housing.

Many women go through these experiences without suffering a depression. But if a woman lacks an intimate relationship with her husband or boyfriend, if she lost her mother through death or divorce before she was eleven, if she has three or more children at home under the age of 14, or if she has no job, then she is more than usually vulnerable to depression. Scoring on more than one of those factors further increases the risk of depression. All these factors, as well as the life events which trigger the depression, involve lack or loss of control over an important area of the woman's life.

Similar considerations apply to women who become depressed when their baby is born. Many feel overwhelmed by the demands of caring for the baby. First-time mothers are obviously at risk here, because our society's ability to prepare them adequately is so pitiful. But post-natal depression tends to recur in the same women, and it can appear for the first time with second or even third babies. These women are likely to feel unable to cope with the demands of the baby and the older children. They may feel very anxious about the baby's progress when by objective standards the baby is thriving. Dr Frederick Melges found that with such mothers the arrival of the baby and the helplessness of the mother can cause the older children to regress and make increased demands on her, creating a vicious circle.[5]

The influence of childhood

A common problem among women who become depressed after birth is the way their own mothers brought them up.[6] Both Melges and Dana Breen found that if a mother is very controlling towards her daughter, the daughter is more likely to become depressed after giving birth. If the mother was also rejecting towards her daughter, then the risk is higher. Both these past experiences involve loss of control. If a mother allows her daughter little initiative in what she does, and at the same time is emotionally cold towards her, the daughter has little control either over the relationship or over her own life. She is unable to establish the contingent responding we described earlier. If a woman lost her mother in childhood she is also at risk.

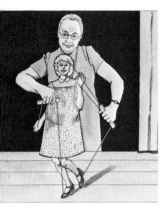

Pregnant puppet on a string? It may depend on how firmly maternal strings are attached.

Lack of support from her husband also makes a woman vulnerable to depression after birth. Some husbands actively dissociate themselves from the birth. Many remain more passively uninvolved, giving neither practical nor emotional support.

Dana Breen found that the women who handle pregnancy and birth best are those who see themselves as active and creative in life generally.

A pair of studies by Eva Frommer and Gillian O'Shea found a more complex picture.[7] A woman whose parents had separated before she was eleven, or who had had a poor relationship with her father or 'father substitute', with the parents quarrelling, was much more likely to be depressed during the pregnancy and after the birth than a woman with a happy and stable home background. A striking finding was that women with unhappy home backgrounds were more likely to have made a special effort to prepare for the coming baby. For some of them, indeed, such preparation led on to a happy and successful motherhood. But among the others, when something went wrong with their environment, marriage or relationship with the baby, then, in the words of Frommer and O'Shea, 'things went more severely awry ... As a group their behaviour tended to polarise into positive and negative aspects.' This is something that it would be as well for both professionals and mothers to bear in mind in cases when a woman does not come up to the expectations she had of herself before the birth.

Depression and the relationship with the baby

Melges also studied the lack of communication which depressed mothers' experience *from* their babies. This may, in fact, be the inability of the mothers to recognise their babies' responses to them. We have seen that babies do respond to their mothers when they are allowed to do so. But the responses are much less definite and much more fleeting than those of adults. A mother needs to treat her baby gently to provoke them and to be sensitive enough to recognise them.

A hospital régime that removes the baby and allows the mother only limited access during feeds is depriving her of the opportunity to establish a relationship in which the baby will respond reliably to her and in which she can recognise the baby's responses.[8] If she is taught that those responses do not exist—as is likely in some places—then her task is made doubly difficult. She is left in a situation where the most important person in her life, her new baby, is out of her reach.

All these factors interact. If the new mother has difficulty in recognising her baby's responses to her, she will tend to feel inadequate as a mother. If she has already effectively been taught that she is inadequate as a woman, and hence as a mother, by her own mother, then her predicament confirms this. If her husband is not able to support her and back her up, her ability as a mother is even further discredited.

Those women who felt either very high or very low levels of anxiety during pregnancy are also more likely than women who felt moderate anxiety to become depressed. Women who respond to pregnancy with very high anxiety are already under stress from a feeling of loss of control. Those who experience low anxiety are denying the reality of their situation. The reality of the birth and the baby come as quite a serious shock, an abrupt change from their preconceived expectations, which is the same as loss of control.

In some women who do not prepare, or are not prepared adequately, for birth, the experience both comes as a shock in itself and is likely to be longer and more painful than average. It removes what Martin Seligman, one of the discoverers of 'learned helplessness', calls the 'safety signal'. Near-misses in accidents can produce terrifying feelings of helplessness and fear in some people, and for a few women their encounter with birth seems to produce the same effect. Again, in such women this effect will interact with others produced by their unpreparedness to cope with the baby.

All these factors are made more powerful if a woman's general home environment and life situation are not very good.

Avoiding depression

Richard and Katherine Gordon have studied ways to help to avoid or clear up post-natal depression.[9] They found that a number of factors involved grouped together to form main factors of conflict with the role of motherhood and personal insecurity. They instituted a programme in which mothers-to-be are instructed and advised on the following points:

> The responsibilities of motherhood are learned: hence *get informed.*
>
> *Get help* from husband and dependable friends and relatives.
>
> *Make friends* of other couples who are experiencing child-rearing.
>
> *Don't overload* yourself with unimportant tasks.
>
> *Don't move* soon after the baby arrives.
>
> *Don't be over-concerned* with keeping up appearances.
>
> Get plenty of *rest and sleep.*
>
> *Don't be a nurse to relatives* and others at this period.
>
> *Confer and consult* with husband, family, and experienced friends, and discuss your plans and worries.
>
> Don't give up outside interests, but *cut down* on responsibilities and rearrange schedules.
>
> Arrange for *baby-sitters* early.
>
> Get a *family doctor*, or see the one you have early.

Women who were given such instruction before birth were much less likely to become depressed or disoriented after birth. Their babies were also less likely to be irritable and to have sleeping and feeding difficulties six months later. If their husbands received the same instruction, the results were even better. Women who had not been given the instruction before birth and had become depressed were helped by receiving the course after the birth.

The effects were also long-lasting. Four to six years later, the mothers who had received the instruction were healthier both physically and mentally than those who had not taken the course. They were also more likely to have had another child. Interestingly, the instruction seems to be more effective if it is given by the woman's own doctor or midwife, rather than as a special course by a psychiatrist.

Other studies have shown that psychotherapy is also effective as a cure if depression develops after birth. Post-natal depression is not usually a physical illness. It is easily understandable, and nearly as easily curable, using the right tools.

Understanding happiness

The psychological factors in pregnancy and birth are still not widely known and many things remain to be discovered. But there is no need for them to be a mystery. The evidence clearly shows that the better a woman understands both the physical and mental changes that occur during the nine months of pregnancy and those that follow, the easier she will find the task she has set herself, and the better she will perform it. To say the same thing in less stern-sounding terms, the more she understands, the happier she, her husband and her baby will be.

I tell ya friends . . .
the result is worth it!

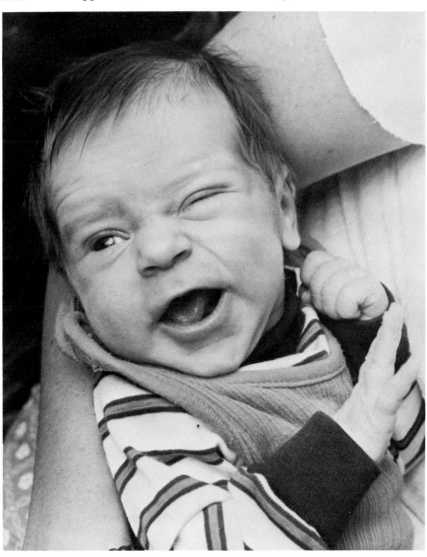

References

1   The background to pregnancy

1. Bowlby, J. *Attachment and Loss, Vol 1: Attachment.* Harmondsworth: Penguin, 1969.
2. Spitz, R. Anaclitic depression. *Psychoanalytic Study of the Child,* 1946, 2, 313–42.
3. Humphrey, M. Sex differences in attitudes to parenthood. *Human Relations,* 1977, 30, 737–49.
4. Gordon, R., & Gordon K. Factors in postpartum emotional adjustment. *Obstetrics and Gynecology,* 1965, 25, 158–66.
5. Laslett, P. The history of population and social structure. *International Social Science Journal,* 1965, 17, 1–12.
6. Deutsch, H. *The Psychology of Women.* London & NY: Grune & Stratton.
7. Donnison, J. *Midwives and Medical Men.* London: Heinemann, 1977.
8. Graham, H. Woman's attitudes to conception and pregnancy. In R. Chester & J. Peel (Eds.). *Equalities and Inequalities in Family Life.* London & NY: Academic Press, 1977.
9. de Mause, Lloyd. *The History of Childhood.* NY: Harper & Row; London: Souvenir Press, 1974.

2   The experience of pregnancy

1. Pohlman, E. *The Psychology of Birth Planning.* Cambridge, Mass.: Schinkman, 1969.
2. Rosenblatt, J. Nonhormonal basis of material behavior in the rat. *Science,* 1967, 156, 1512–3.
3. Hinde, R. A., & McGinnis, L. Some factors influencing the effects of temporary mother-infant separation: some experiments with rhesus monkeys. *Psychological Medicine,* 1977, 7, 197–212.
4. de Beauvoir, S. *The Second Sex.* NY: Random. Harmondsworth: Penguin, 1968.
5. Leifer, M. Psychological changes in pregnancy. *Genetic Psychology Monographs,* 1977, 95, 55–96.
6. Anon. *You and Your Baby.* Family Doctor Publications, 1975.
7. Caplan, G. *An Approach to Community Mental Health.* London & Chicago: Grune & Stratton, 1961.
8. Chapple, P. A. L., & Furneaux, W. D. Changes in personality and labour. *Proceedings of the Royal Society of Medicine,* 1964, 57, 260–1.
9. King, F. T. *Feeding and Baby Care,* 1921.
10. Busfield, J., & Paddon, M. *Thinking about Children.* Cambridge: CUP, 1977.
11. Rainwater, L. *Family Design: Marital Sexuality, Family Size and Contraception.* Chicago: Aldine Press, 1965.
12. Benedek, T. Parenthood as a developmental phase. *Journal of the American Psychoanalytic Association,* 1959, 7, 389–417.
13. Bibring, G. A study of the psychological processes in pregnancy and of the earliest mother-child relationship. *Psychoanalytic Study of the Child,* 1961, 16, 9–72.
14. de Beauvoir, S. op. cit.

15. Busfield, J. & Paddon, M. op. cit.
16. Leifer, M. op. cit.

4   Adapting to pregnancy

1. Rubin, R. Attainment of the maternal role, Pt. I: Processes. *Nursing Research,* 1967, 16, 237–45. Pt 2: Models and Referrants. *Nursing Research,* 1967, 16, 342–6.
2. Graham, H. Personal communication.
3. Rubin, R. op. cit.
4. Graham, H. Personal communication.
5. Lumley, J. The development of maternal-fetal bonding in first pregnancy. (Paper delivered at 5th World Congress on Psychosomatic Medicine in Obstetrics and Gynaecology.)
6. Lumley, J. op. cit.

5   Emotions in pregnancy

1. Graham, H. *Images of Pregnancy.* (Unpublished Mimeograph.)
2. Smith, S. L. Mood and the Menstrual Cycle. In E. J. Sacher (Ed.), *Topics in Psychoendocrinology.* London & Chicago: Grune & Stratton, 1975.
3. Paige, K. E. Women learn to sing the menstrual blues. *Psychology Today,* 1973, US Edn., 7, 4:41–46. (In UK Edn., as The Curse on Women, 1973, 1, 2:36.)
4. Smith, S. L. op. cit.
5. Asso, D., & Beech, H. R. Susceptibility to the acquisition of a conditioned response in relation to the menstrual cycle. *Journal of Psychosomatic Research,* 1975, 19, 337–44.
6. Vila, J., & Beech, H. R. Vulnerability and defensive reactions to the menstrual cycle. *British Journal of Social and Clinical Psychology,* 1978, 17, 93–100.
7. Lubin, B., et al. Mood and somatic symptoms during pregnancy. *Psychosomatic Medicine,* 1975, 37, 136–46.
8. Cramond, W. A. Psychological aspects of uterine dysfunction. *Lancet,* 1974, 11, Dec, 1242–5.
9. Graham, H. The social image of pregnancy: Pregnancy as spirit possession. *Sociological Review,* 1976, 24, 291–308.
10. Rosengren, W. R. Social sources of pregnancy as illness or normality. *Social Forces,* 1961a, 39, 260–7. Some psychological aspects of delivery room difficulties. *Journal of Mental and Nervous Diseases,* 1961b, 132, 515–21.
11. Douglas, G. Puerperal depression and excessive compliance with the mother. *British Journal of Medical Psychology,* 1963, 36, 271–8.
12. Meyerowitz, J. H., & Feldman, H. Transition to Parenthood. *Psychiatric Research Reports,* 1966, 20, 78–94.
13. Baum, M. Love, marriage and the division of labour. In H. P. Dreitzel (Ed.), *Family, Marriage and the Struggle of the Sexes.* NY: Macmillan, 1972.
14. Goshen-Gottenstein, E. *Marriage and First Pregnancy: Cultural Influences on Attitudes of Israeli Woman.* Philidelphia: Lippincott, 1966.

6   The body and sex in pregnancy

1. Adams, D. B., et al. Rise in female initiated sexual activity at ovulation and its suppression by oral contraceptives. *New England Journal of Medicine,* 1978, 229, 1145–50.
2. Sandler, B. Emotional stress and infertility. *Journal of Psychonomic Research,* 1968, 12, 51–9.
3. Heiman, J. Lady's relish. *Psychology Today,* 1975, UK Edit., 1, 4, 57–60.

4. Bardwick, J., & Behrman, S. J. Investigation into the effects of anxiety, sexual arousal and menstrual cycle phase on uterine contractions. *Psychonomic Medicine,* 1967, 29, 486–82

5. Baxter, S. Orgasm and labour in primiparae. *Journal of Psychonomic Research,* 1974, 18, 357–60.

6. Fisher, S. *Understanding the Female Orgasm.* NY: Basic Books; Harmondsworth: Penguin, 1973.

7. Tolor, A., & di Grazia, P. V. Sexual attitudes and behaviour during and following pregnancy. *Archives of Sexual Behavior,* 1976, 5, 539–51.

8. Masters, W., & Johnson, V. *Human Sexual Response.* Boston: Little Brown, 1966.

9. Meyerowitz, J. H., & Feldman, H. Transition to Parenthood. *Psychiatric Research Reports,* 1966, 20, 78–94.

10. Shereshefsky, P. M. & Yarrow, L.J. (Eds.), *Psychological Aspects of a First Pregnancy and Early Postnatal Adaption.* NY: Raven Press, 1973.

11. Solberg, D. A., et al. Sexual Behaviour in Pregnancy. *New England Journal of Medicine,* 1973, May, 1098–1103.

12. Hollander, M. H., & McGhee, J. B. The wish to be held during pregnancy. *Journal of Psychonomic Research,* 1974, 18, 193–7.

13. Bardwick, J. *Readings on the Psychology of Women.* NY: Harper & Row.

14. Hollender, M., et al. Body contact and sexual excitement. *Archives of General Psychiatry,* 1969, 20, 188–91.

7   Fathers in pregnancy and birth

1. Lamb, M. E. (Ed.), *The Role of the Father in Infant Development.* NY: Wiley, 1976.

2. Wainwright, W. H. Fatherhood as a precipitant of mental illness. *American Journal of Psychiatry,* 1966, 123, 40–44.

3. Curtiss, J. L. A psychiatric study of 55 expectant fathers. *United States Armed Forces Medical Journal,* 1955, 6, 937–50.

4. Hartman, A. A., & Nicolay, R. C. Sexually deviant behavior in expectant fathers. *Journal of Abnormal Psychology,* 1966, 71, 232–4.

5. George, V., & Wilding, P. *Motherless Families.* London & Boston: Routledge & Kegan Paul, 1972.

6. Coley, S. B., & James, B. E. Delivery: a trauma for fathers? *The Family Co-ordinator,* 1976, 25, 359–63.

7. Cavenar, J. O., & Butts, N. T. Fatherhood and emotional illness. *American Journal of Psychiatry,* 1977, 134, 429–31.

8. Barry, W. A. Marriage research and conflict: an integrative review. *Psychological Bulletin,* 1970, 73, 41–54.

9. Wenner, N. K., et al. Emotional problems in pregnancy. *Psychiatry,* 1969, 32, 389–410.

10. Zajicek, E., & Wolkind, S. Emotional difficulties in married women during and after the first pregnancy. *British Journal of Medical Psychology* (in press).

11. Overton, I. M. K. The development of neuroses in the wives of neurotic men. *British Journal of Medical Psychology,* 1973, 122, 35–45.

12. Lumley, J. The development of maternal-fetal bonding in first pregnancy. (Paper delivered at 5th World Congress on Psychosomatic Obstetrics and Gynaecology).

13. Greenberg, M., & Morris, N. Engrossment: the newborns' impact upon the father. *American Journal of Orthopsychiatry,* 1974, 44, 520–31.

14. Gayton, R. *A Comparison of Natural and Non-natural Childbirth Fathers.* (Unpublished PhD Thesis, US International University).

15. Bradley, R. A. *Husband Coached Childbirth.* NY: Harper & Row, 1965.

16. Huttell, F. A., et al. A quantitative evaluation of psychoprophylaxis in childbirth. *Journal of Psychonomic Res.*, 1972, 16, 81–92.

8 Problems in pregnancy

1. Chertok, L. Vomiting and the wish to have a child. *Psychosomatic Medicine*, 1963, 25, 13–18.
2. Wolkind, S., & Zajicek, E. Psycho-social correlates of nausea and vomiting in pregnancy. *J. Psychosomatic Research*, 1978, 22, 1–5.
3. Uddenberg, N., et al. Nausea in pregnancy: psychological and psychosomatic aspects. *J. Psychonomic Research*, 1971, 15, 269–76.
4. Coppen, A. J., et al. Vomiting of early pregnancy: psychological factors and body build. *Lancet*, 1959, 1, 172.
5. Hetzel, B. S., et al. A survey of the relation between certain common antenatal complications in primiparae and stressful life situations during pregnancy. *J. Psychonomic Research*, 1961, 5, 172–82.
6. Hetzel, B. S., et al., ibid.
7. McDonald, R. L. The role of emotional factors in obstetric complications: a review. *Psychosomatic Medicine*, 1968, 30, 222–35.

9 Preparing for birth: pain and childbirth classes

1. Garrey, M. M., et al. *Obstetrics Illustrated.* Edinburgh: Churchill Livingstone. NY: Longman, 1974.
2. Read, G. D. *Natural Childbirth.* London: Heinemann, 1933.
3. Trethowan, W. H., & Conlon, M. F. The Couvade Syndrome. *British Journal of Psychiatry*, 1965, 111, 57–66.
4. Murray, J. B. Psychology of the pain experience. *Psychology*, 1971, 78, 193.
5. Melzack, R. *The Puzzle of Pain.* Harmondsworth: Penguin. NY: Basic Books, 1973.
6. Beecher, H. K. The measurement of pain. *Pharmacological Review*, 1957, 9, 59.
7. Eysenck, S. B. G. Personality and pain assessment in childbirth of married and unmarried mothers. *Journal of Mental Science*, 1961, 107, 417–30.
8. Andrew, J. Coping style, stress-relevant learning and recovery from surgery. *Dissertion Abstracts*, 1968, 1182–B.
9. Almgren, P. E., et al. Psykologiska faktorer vid forlossning. *Sartyck ur Lakertidningen*, 1972, 69, 3126.
10. Davidson, P. O. (Ed.), *The Behavioral Management of Anxiety, Depression and Pain.* NY: Brunner Mazel, 1976.
11. Bobey, M. J., & Davidson, P. O. Psychological factors affecting pain tolerance. *J. Psychosomatic Research*, 1970, 14, 371–76.
12. Stevens, R. J., & Heide, F. Analgesic characteristics of prepared childbirth techniques: attention focussing and systematic relaxation. *J. Psychosomatic Research*, 1977, 21, 429–38.
13. Enkin, M., et al. An adequately controlled study of the effectiveness of PPM training. In N. Morris (Ed.), *Psychosomatic Medicine in Obstetrics and Gynaecology.* White Plains, NY: Karger.
14. Huttell, F. A., et al. A quantitative evaluation of psychoprophylaxis in childbirth. *J. Psychonomic Research*, 1972, 19, 215–222.
15. Doering, S. G. & Entwisle, D. R. Preparation during pregnancy and ability to cope with labour and delivery. *American Journal of Orthopsychiatry*, 1975, 45, 825–37.

10 Mother and baby

1. McGurk, H. Visual perception in young infants. In B. Foss (Ed.), *New Perspectives in Child Development.* NY & Harmondsworth: Penguin, 1974.

2. Packer, M. & Rosenblatt, D. Issues in the study of social behavior in the first week of life. In J. Dunn., & D. Schaffer (Eds.), *The First Year of Life.* NY: Wiley, 1978.

3. Ciba Foundation. *Parent-Infant Interaction.* Amsterdam: Elsevier, 1975.

4. Mills, M., & Melhuish, E. Recognition of mother's voice in early infancy. *Nature,* 1974, 252, 123–4.

5. Carpenter, G. Mother's face and the newborn. *New Scientist,* 1974, 21st March, 742–4.

6. Sander, L. W. Regulation and organisation in the early infant-caretaker system. In R. J. Robinson (Ed.), *Brain and Early Behavior.* London & NY: Academic Press, 1969.

7. Richards, M. P. M. Effects on infant behavior of analgesics and anaesthetics used in obstetrics. (Paper presented at 5th conference of the European Teratology Society, 1976).

8. Rutter, M. *Maternal Deprivation Reassessed.* NY & Harmondsworth: Penguin, 1972.

9. Newton, N. Psychologic differences between breast and bottle feeding. *American Journal of Clinical Nutrition,* 1971, 24, 993–1004.

10. Klaus, M. H., & Kennel, J. H. *Maternal–Infant Bonding.* St. Louis, MO.: Mosby, 1976.

11. Whiten, A. In M. P. M. Richards., & F. S. W. Brimblecomb, (Eds.), *Early Separation and Special Care Nurseries.* London: Heinemann, 1978.

12. Jelliffe, D. B., & Jelliffe, E. F. P. *Human Milk in the Modern World.* Oxford: OUP, 1978.

13. Escalona, S. K. Feeding disturbances in very young children. *American Journal of Orthopsychiatry,* 1945, 15, 76–80.

14. De Chateau, P., et al. A study of factors promoting and inhibiting lactation. *Developmental Medicine and Child Neurology,* 1977, 19, 575–84.

11 Depression and the blues

1. Pitt, B. A typical depression following childbirth. *British Journal of Psychiatry,* 1968b, 114, 1325–35.

2. Hamilton, J. A. *Postpartum psychiatric syndromes.* St. Louis, Mo.: Mosby, 1962.

3. Seligman, M. *Helplessness: on Depression, Development and Death.* San Francisco & Reading: Freeman, 1975.

4. Brown, G. G., et al. *Social Origins of Depression.* London: Tavistock, 1978.

5. Melges, F. T. Postpartum psychiatric syndromes. *Psychosomatic Medicine,* 1968, 30, 95–108.

6. Douglas, G. Puerperal depression and excessive compliance with the mother. *British Journal of Medical Psychology,* 1963, 36, 271–8.

7. Frommer, E. A., & O'Shea, G. Antenatal identification of woman liable to have problems with managing their infants. *British Journal of Psychiatry,* 1973a, 123, 149–56. The importance of childhood experience in relation to problems of marriage and family building. *British Journal of Psychiatry,* 1973b, 123, 157–60.

8. Robinson, J. How hospitals alienate mothers. *Mind Out,* 1976, March/April, 7–9.

9. Gordon, R. E., Kapostins, E. E., & Gordon, K. K. Factors in postpartum emotional adjustment. *Obstetrics and Gynecology,* 1965, 25, 158–66.

Suggested further reading

Antony, A. J., & Benedek, T. *Parenthood: its Psychology and Psychopathology.* Boston: Little Brown. Edinburgh: Churchill Livingstone, 1970.

Bardwick, J. M. *Psychology of Women.* NY: Harper & Row, 1971.

Breen, D. *The Birth of the First Child.* London: Tavistock, 1974.

Kitzinger, S. *Giving Birth: the Parents' Emotions in Childbirth.* London: Gollancz, NY: Taplinger, 1971. *Education and Counselling for Childbirth.* London: Bailliere Tindall, 1977. *The Experience of Childbirth.* NY & Harmondsworth: Penguin, 1978 (4th Edition).

Money, J., & Musaph, H. *Handbook of Sexology.* Amsterdam: Elsevier, 1977.

Rapoport, R., Rapoport, R. N., & Strelitz, Z. *Fathers, Mothers and Others.* London & Boston: Routledge, Kegan Paul, 1977.

Richards, M. P. M. (Ed.), *The Integration of the Child into a Social World.* Cambridge: CUP, 1974.

Shereshefsky, P. M., & Yarrow, L. J. (Eds.), *Psychological Aspects of a First Pregnancy and Early Postnatal Adaption.* NY: Raven Press, 1973.

Index

Acknowledgments

Many people have contributed, directly and indirectly, to the creation of this book; too many to mention everyone. Christopher Macy wishes to record his special thanks for help and encouragement at the outset to Nicholas Blurton-Jones and his team; to Eva Zajicek and Fae Hall of the Family Research Unit, London Hospital; to Hilary Graham of the University of York; to Deborah Rosenblatt of the Perinatal Research Unit of St. Mary's Hospital, London; and to Leonard Kristal of Multimedia Publications Inc.

The authors pay special tribute to the definitive research of Reva Rubin and Myra Leifer, of Robert Fein and Richard Gayton, of Hilary Graham and Sally Macintyre, and of the Medical Psychology Unit at the University of Cambridge, particularly the contributions of Martin Richards and Judy Bernal Dunn.

Photo credits

Michael Abrahams—74; Aliza Auerbach—9 (*top*; *bottom*), 84; Frank Bez (Rex)—68; Bob Bray—24 (*right*), 27, 31, 33, 44, 108; Werner Braun—80, 105; Marcus Brooke (Colorific)—41 (*right*); Ben Card—36 (*top*); Camera Press—89, 90, 91; G. V. P. Chamberlain MD, FRCS, FRCOG—45; Ron Chapman—26; John Cleare—51; Dorothy Perkins—6; M. Garanger (Rex)—76; Ya'acov Harlap—62, 107, 111; David Harris—12; Prof. Dr. Heinz Kirchhoff—14, 15 (*top*; *middle*; *bottom*), 92, 94, 101; Judy Kristal—109; C. Leimbach—71; Mary Evans Picture Library—22; Mothercare—36 (*bottom*), 46, 99; Margaret Murray—10; Paf International—24 (*left*), 39, 42, 47, 55, 119; Colin Poole—56; Rex Features—8, 11 (*centre*; *right*), 13, 19, 20, 23 (*left*), 29, 58, 59, 61, 65, 73, 86, 112; Robert Harding—5; Anthea Sieveking—37, 41 (*left*), 77, 96, 97, 104, 106; Clark Sunida & Bob Harvey Globe Photos (Rex)—11 (*left*), 23, 78; Homer Sykes—57; Tony Stone—16; Valerie Wilmer—102.